The
Antioxidant
Health Plan

The
Antioxidant
Health Plan
HOW TO BEAT
THE EFFECTS OF
FREE RADICALS

———❖———

Dr Robert Youngson

Thorsons
An Imprint of HarperCollins*Publishers*

Thorsons
An Imprint of HarperCollins*Publishers*
77—85 Fulham Palace Road
Hammersmith, London W6 8JB
1160 Battery Street
San Francisco, California 94111—1213

Published by Thorsons 1994
10 9 8 7 6 5 4 3 2 1

A catalogue record for this book
is available from the British Library

ISBN 0 7225 2968 6

Phototypeset by Harper Phototypesetters Limited,
Northampton, England
Printed in Great Britain by
HarperCollinsManufacturing Glasgow

Contents

Introduction

Linus Pauling, twice a Nobel Prize winner and now 92 years old, is one of the most distinguished scientists of the century. His book *The Nature of the Chemical Bond and the Structure of Molecules and Crystals* revolutionized chemistry and has been described as one of the most influential science texts ever written. He played a major part in laying the foundations of modern chemistry, biochemistry and molecular biology. He adapted chemistry to quantum mechanics and pioneered several fundamental methods of determining molecular structure. *New Scientist* described him as one of the 20 greatest scientists of all time, on a par with Newton, Darwin and Einstein. Most people would agree that Pauling is no fool.

In 1970 Pauling published a book called *Vitamin C and the Common Cold* in which he expressed the opinion, based on careful observation of his own experience, that regular daily dosage of this vitamin, in amounts well in excess of the minimum required to prevent deficiency, would produce '. . . an increased feeling of wellbeing, and especially a striking decrease in the number of colds caught, and in their severity'. Pauling examined previous trials of the method, most of which had produced disappointing results, and pointed out that the dosage that had been given in these trials was nowhere near large enough. But in spite of his persuasive arguments, he was dismissed by many of his colleagues as a crank.

That is how matters stood for ten years or so, and then the unexpected happened. Something new and very important quietly emerged in medicine — nothing less than an understanding of the way human cells, tissues and organs are damaged, not only in minor disorders like the common cold, but also in major conditions like heart disease and cancer, and even in ageing. The literature on this subject in the medical journals has been growing steadily, but in the last two or three years it has suddenly erupted. Many hundreds of papers have now been published in journals like *The Lancet*, the *British Medical Journal*, the *New England Journal of Medicine* and the *Journal of the American Medical Association*. The interest has been so great that there has even been at least one completely new journal devoted exclusively to the subject. The general scientific journals like *Nature* and *Science*, the specialized biochemical and molecular biology journals, and the popular science magazines like *New Scientist* and *Scientific American* have also published widely in this area.

All these original papers and reviews indicate that this vital tissue damage is caused by microscopic groups of chemicals, known as *free radicals*, which are naturally produced in enormous numbers in the body. Free radicals also occur in cigarette smoke, car exhaust and industrial fumes, and are generated in the body when it is exposed to ultraviolet light from the sun and other forms of radiation. Produced in excess and not checked, the destructive effect of free radicals on body cells and thus on many tissues and organs can be very serious. Their role in the causation of the arterial disease atherosclerosis, that leads to most cases of heart disease and other serious conditions such as gangrene, is now well understood. Atherosclerosis, incidentally, is the number one killer in the Western world, and claims more victims than any other single cause. The damaging effect of free radicals on the heart muscle after a heart attack is also clear. An enormous amount of research has shown that free radical damage is implicated in a wide range of other diseases and disorders. These include:

- Coronary thrombosis
- Angina pectoris
- Heart failure
- Stroke
- Brain damage
- Ageing
- Kidney disease
- Cancer
- Inflammatory disorders
- Cataract
- Poisoning
- Radiation sickness
- Rheumatoid arthritis
- Male infertility
- Retinopathy of prematurity
- Malnutrition

This discovery alone is a major medical advance that has already begun to have an important impact on the understanding of disease processes. But this is not all. There is now strong and increasing evidence that the damaging effects of excess free radicals *can be limited or even prevented* by taking large doses of *antioxidant* substances such as vitamin C and vitamin E. Beta-carotene, the antioxidant provitamin A, has also been shown to be an important weapon against free radicals. Beta-carotene is the stuff that makes carrots orange and is converted by the liver into vitamin A.

To quote biochemistry Professor A. T. Diplock of Guy's and St Thomas's hospitals, London:

Compelling evidence is now emerging from prospective studies begun in the early 1970s that low dietary intake of vitamin E is indeed a significant risk factor in the aetiogenesis of both ischaemic heart disease and cancer at certain sites. Several prospective studies have shown a correlation between a low dietary level of vitamin C and a high incidence of cardiovascular disease and cancer. Strong prospective epidemiological evidence now emerging implies a close correlation between a high level of serum beta-carotene and a low incidence of cancer. These correlations have been particularly strong for lung cancer.

Translated into ordinary language, this means that scientific trials have proved that people who don't take enough vitamin E and vitamin C are more likely to get heart attacks and certain kinds of cancers. People who take enough provitamin A are less likely to get cancer, especially lung cancer.

Free radicals do their damage by a common chemical process known as oxidation. No one now questions that antioxidant substances can 'mop up' free radicals and prevent them from damaging cells. Vitamin C is one of the best known and most effective biological antioxidants, so it really does begin to look as if Linus Pauling might have been right after all.

Already the subject of free radicals is getting to be big news outside scientific circles. Essential facts that scientists have known for several years are gradually coming together to form a picture that may well transform medicine, and these facts are beginning to filter through to non-scientists.

I have been watching these developments closely for about five years now and it seems to me that the time has come to spread the news more widely. This is why I have decided to write this book, to put the facts before you, without any attempt at a 'hard sell', so that you can make up your own mind. I have had to dig out the facts from a mass of research reports, but have tried to present them in as non-technical and accessible language as possible. I have no doubt about the importance of this remarkable advance in medical knowledge; now I am challenging you to find out what it is all about.

Read on.

What are Free Radicals?

Free radicals are dangerous. They can do you a lot of harm. If your body fails to combat them effectively, they will kill you. We now know that most of the major diseases that kill people prematurely or ruin the quality of life do their damage by means of free radicals. They are constantly attacking body proteins, carbohydrates, fats and DNA, causing potentially serious damage unless checked. Every cell in your body suffers an estimated 10,000 free radical hits each day. The body strikes back, as we shall see. This is a real battlefield.

There is no way you can avoid free radicals, but there is a lot you can do to cut down the numbers produced in your body and to ensure that the maximum number of those that *are* produced are neutralized. How can this be done? In this chapter I shall outline the basic scientific facts underlying the whole matter. Unless you know a little about science, you may find it difficult in places, for a subject like this cannot be adequately covered without a few technicalities. However, I recommend that you work through it — and hope that it may not be that bad, after all! Then you will not only be able to read the rest of this book with a clearer understanding, but also be able to take a more critical and intelligent interest in future newspaper and magazine articles on the subject.

The Chemists and the Radicals

Medical interest in free radicals is very recent, but chemists have been studying them closely for about 50 years. When they were first proposed about 100 years ago, most chemists were outraged and protested that they were impossible. Gradually, however, they came to realize that free radicals were very real and were fleetingly involved in many important chemical reactions, such as the formation of plastics (polymers), the perishing of rubber and the deterioration of stored foodstuffs. Most free radicals exist only for very short periods before attacking other substances and being neutralized in the process. They can, however, be produced as quickly as they disappear and when they do attack they can turn other substances into free radicals and set up very damaging chain reactions.

So, what are they?

Atoms

Everything is made of atoms. One free radical consists of a single atom, others of two atoms linked together. Those that we are mainly interested in each consist of two atoms linked together. But these are not ordinary atoms. They are atoms with one very special property that makes all the difference to their significance to us. To make this plain, we must take a brief look at atoms in general.

Every atom has a central part, called the *nucleus*, and a number of tiny particles, called *electrons*, buzzing around it. That's all. The rest is empty space. A vacuum. The nucleus is charged positive and the electrons are charged negative, and there are the same number of electrons as there are positive charges on the nucleus. So the atom, as a whole, has no charge because all the positive charges are neutralized by the negative charges. The electrons occupy regions around the nucleus known as *orbitals*. Each orbital can hold only two electrons and these are spinning in opposite directions. An orbital with two electrons is stable; an orbital with only one electron is highly unstable.

Atoms differ in the number of electrons they have. There are 92 different kinds of atom in nature, from hydrogen, the lightest, to uranium, the heaviest, and scientists have made a dozen more. Substances made of collections of atoms of one kind only are called elements. So there are 92 natural elements. Hydrogen has one electron; uranium has 92. So hydrogen has a problem. With only one electron, how does it achieve a stable, two-electron orbital? It solves this problem very quickly, simply by linking up with another hydrogen atom to form a pair that share a filled, two-electron orbital.

Molecules

Most substances are made from a combination of different kinds of atoms linked together. These combinations of atoms are called *molecules*. They may be quite small or very large. The molecule of hydrogen consists of two hydrogen atoms linked together. Molecules may contain a few atoms or many. Molecules of proteins or plastics are very large and may contain hundreds, thousands or even millions of atoms, usually of just a few varieties, all linked together.

Substances made of molecules are called *compounds* and most of these contain just a few different kinds of atoms. Water, for instance consists of an oxygen atom linked to two hydrogen atoms: H_2O. Common salt consists of an atom of the metal sodium linked to an atom of the gas chlorine: $NaCl$. Human beings are made from just over 20 different atoms, but 93.3 per cent of our bodies are made from only four — carbon, hydrogen, oxygen and nitrogen.

Atomic Bonds

When atoms bond to each other to form molecules they do so by sharing their outer electrons in various ways. These linkages are called *bonds*. Some atoms can link to only one other atom; some can link to two; some to three; some to four. A single atom of the element carbon can link to four other atoms, including other carbon atoms and this is why the chemistry of carbon is a complete science in its own right, known as organic chemistry. Carbon atoms can link together in long chains, with other kinds of atoms hooked on, or they can link together in rings of six atoms (benzene rings) or in different-sized rings with other atoms. The permutations are almost infinite.

If a carbon atom links to fewer than the full number of atoms it is capable of linking to, it forms double, or even triple, bonds. These are *weaker* than single bonds, because the carbon atom likes to have all its four bonds properly used up. Compounds with double bonds are said to be *unsaturated*; those with only single bonds are *saturated*.

Organic Molecules and Chemical Groups

Most organic molecules — those found in living things or their products — are fairly large. All of them are based on carbon and many consists of only carbon and hydrogen, or carbon, hydrogen and oxygen, linked up in chains or rings. Most organic molecules consist of a kind of basic structure of carbon atoms to which small clusters of other atoms are attached. These clusters, or chemical *groups*, are very important in chemistry, especially in biochemistry — the chemistry of living things — as different groups are responsible for most of the different chemical properties of the molecules.

4

In 1832 the German chemists Baron von Liebig and Friedrich Wöhler discovered that, when chemical reactions occurred, these little clusters, instead of breaking up to release the individual atoms of which they are made, tended to act almost like molecules in their own right, retaining their group identity and linking on, in their entirety, to other molecules. They did not, however, persist for any length of time on their own but always tried to tie themselves on to a molecule. It was decided to call these groups *radicals*. This word has no deep hidden meaning. It simply comes from the Latin word *radix*, meaning 'a root', and was selected because the atom cluster hangs from the molecule like a root and can 'root' itself in other molecules.

As you may have guessed, *free radicals* are radicals that are temporarily unattached to a molecule. Unattached radicals are not happy just to sit around like the more stable molecules of compounds; rather they are constantly looking for something to latch on to. Many of them are quite small, consisting of only two or three atoms; some are larger. The one thing they all have in common is that they are remarkably active — and some of them are highly dangerous to our bodies.

Ions and Ionization

As we have seen, water consists of a single atom of oxygen with two hydrogen atoms linked on to it. The bonds between the oxygen atom and each hydrogen atom consist of a pair of electrons shared between the atoms — one from the hydrogen atom and one from the oxygen atom. The water molecule, however, routinely separates into two particles, one consisting of a hydrogen atom without its electron (H) and the other consisting of a hydrogen atom linked to the oxygen atom (OH). Because the nucleus of an atom is positively charged and the electrons are negative, a hydrogen atom without its electron carries a positive charge (H +). Such a particle is called a positive *ion* (the term comes from a Greek word meaning 'wanderer'). The missing electron is stuck on to the oxygen/hydrogen combination (OH) which, with the extra electron is thus a negative ion (OH-). Because it contains a hydrogen and an oxygen atom it is called a *hydroxyl ion*. This is the normal way for water to be split up and is known as *ionization*. Positive and negative ions are important in chemistry, and many chemical reactions occur between different ions coming together.

The Unpaired Electron

About 50 years ago it was discovered — to the astonishment of the chemists — that, under certain circumstances, the water molecule can split up in another, quite different, way. If, for instance, water is exposed to radiation such as X-rays or gamma rays, the two-electron bonds between the oxygen and the hydrogen atoms can briefly split, leaving one electron on the hydrogen and one on the oxygen, thus creating two radicals, both electrically neutral but both having only one spare electron. Thus, momentarily, we have two atoms each with only one electron in an outer orbital. These radicals are known, respectively, as the *hydrogen radical* and the *hydroxyl radical*, and both of them are horribly active. The hydroxyl radical is the most reactive free radical known to chemistry and will attack almost every molecule in the body.

It is the unpaired electron that makes these radicals so chemically active. A group with an unpaired electron is highly unstable and is desperate either to pick up another electron from somewhere, or to give up its solitary electron.

Nature likes things to be stable. Hydrogen atoms, which have only one electron, never exist individually for more than a fraction of a second, but immediately join up in pairs to produce a hydrogen molecule of two atoms with a stable pair of electrons (H_2). The same applies to a hydrogen radical — which is, of course, simply an isolated hydrogen atom. It is this stable state that free radicals are always aiming for, and if a free radical is formed, it will at once attack the nearest molecule — whatever it may be — in order to steal or hand over an electron and achieve stability. This can have very serious effects.

So now we have a definition of a free radical. A free radical is *any atom or group of atoms that can exist independently and that contains at least one unpaired electron*. Some free radicals exist for appreciable lengths of time. But the great majority have only a very brief independent existence before either grabbing an extra electron or giving one up. Not all free radicals are small, like the hydrogen or hydroxyl radicals. The methyl radical has a carbon atom and three hydrogen atoms; the ethyl radical has two carbons and five hydrogens. Some are large and complex, containing rings of carbon atoms (benzene rings) and various side chains. All however, have a single, unpaired, electron somewhere.

Free Radical Chain Reactions

From the medical point of view we are interested mainly in two free radicals: the *hydroxyl radical* (-OH) and the *superoxide radical*, which consists of two linked oxygen atoms ($O_2 \cdot$) with a single, unpaired electron.

These oxygen free radicals, each with their single electron, can attack and damage almost every molecule found in the body. They are so active that, after they are formed, only a small fraction of a second elapses before they join on to something. In so doing they can either hand over their unpaired electron or capture an electron from some other molecule to make up the pair. In either event the radicals become stable but *the attacked molecule is, itself, converted into a radical*. This starts a chain reaction that can zip destructively through a tissue.

Free radical action is not, of course, limited to the human body. but occurs throughout all chemistry. Many plastics are made by the free radical action that breaks double carbon bonds and allows small chemical units (*monomers*) to be joined repeatedly in a long chain to form a *polymer*. (*Poly* is the Greek word for 'many'.) Polythene, for instance, is made by a free radical chain reaction to link up many ethene monomers. Synthetic rubber is made in a similar way. Even paint drying involves free radical reactions.

Radiation and Chain Reactions

In living systems, the hydroxyl free radical does not normally occur, because of the strength of the bonds holding the water molecules together. But if anyone is exposed to radiation, these bonds can be broken by the radiation so that hydroxyl radicals result. This is the basis of the dreadful, often fatal, damage that occurs in people with radiation sickness. If hydroxyl radicals attack DNA, chain reactions run along the DNA molecule causing damage to, and mutations in, the genetic material or even actual breakage of the DNA strands. The body does its best to repair this damage by the natural processes of DNA replication, but imperfect repair leaves altered DNA and can give rise to cancer. When strong X- and gamma radiation is deliberately used to kill cancers, it does so primarily by producing large numbers of hydroxyl free radicals.

Radiation is not the only way free radicals are produced, and free radicals are not only produced from water. But radiation is the only common way that hydroxyl free radicals are formed in the body *from water*. Unfortunately, there are other ways in which hydroxyl radicals can be formed and there are several other kinds of free radicals, especially the superoxide radical, that can be produced in other ways. They are produced by many disease processes, by poisons, drugs, metals, cigarette smoke, car exhausts, heat, lack of oxygen, even by sunlight. There is much more about this in later chapters.

Oxidation

In general terms, the damage that is done by free radicals features the chemical reaction known as *oxidation* and free radical attacks on tissue is known as *oxidative stress*. This idea of oxidation is particularly important and deserves a closer look.

If a bright iron nail is left outside it will soon rust. If you strike a match and let it burn, the firm white wood turns to a brittle, blackened ash. If you start your car, a little petrol gets turned to a mixture of gases and soot that come out of the exhaust pipe. These are all examples of the common chemical change known as oxidation. In all these cases the element oxygen — which makes up about 20 per cent of the atmospheric air — links up chemically with the original substance, whether iron, cellulose or hydrocarbon, to form an entirely new compound. If the nail rusts completely — which it will eventually do if exposed to air and water — it turns to a pile of red powdery stuff called iron oxide. When the match and the petrol are oxidized, equally major changes occur in which the carbon, hydrogen and oxygen of which they are made combine with oxygen from the air to form new compounds. These are mostly gases — water vapour (hydrogen and oxygen) and carbon dioxide (carbon and oxygen). The ash of the match and the soot from the exhaust are mostly carbon that has not linked with oxygen to form carbon dioxide.

The whole point about striking matches and burning petrol is to release energy. Oxidation is always associated with a release of energy, usually in the form of heat. Even the rusting of the nail releases heat, but very slowly, so we don't usually notice it. The heat from the match is obvious, and that from the petrol expands the gas in the cylinders of the car engine, drives down the pistons and moves the car along. When you eat a McDonald's cheeseburger, it too is oxidized — rather slowly so that the heat energy is released at a suitable rate to keep up your body temperature and supply energy to the cells.

Releasing energy is always a double-edged weapon. So, although oxidation is obviously important and necessary, it can also be damaging. Matches can light the gas, but they can also set fire to a house. Petrol and other active or explosive substances can be used in different ways when they are oxidized, some constructive, some destructive. It is exactly the same with free radicals. The body can't do without them, because they are involved in many essential chemical reactions. But if more free radicals are produced than the body needs, or if the body's methods of coping with free radicals prove inadequate, then we are in trouble.

Although the term oxidation originally meant adding oxygen, as in these examples, it has now been extended to have a wider meaning. Chemists now define oxidation as any chemical reaction that involves the loss of an electron from an atom. And, as we have seen, removing electrons from atoms is exactly what free radicals are particularly good at doing.

How Are Oxygen Free Radicals Produced in the Body?

Free radicals can originate in body cells in various ways. External radiation, including ultraviolet light, X-rays and gamma rays from radioactive material, is a potent source. Such radiation acts by breaking linkages between atoms, leaving the radicals with their unpaired electrons to wreak their damage. Free radicals occur in the course of various disease processes. In a heart attack, for instance, when the supply of oxygen and glucose to the heart muscle is cut off, the real damage to the muscle is caused by the vast numbers of free radicals that are produced.

Chemical poisoning of many kinds promotes free radicals, as does excessive oxygen intake from inhaling pure oxygen. The body's necessity to break down a wide range of drugs to safer substances (detoxication) also involves free radical production. The poisonousness (toxicity) of many chemicals and drugs is actually due either to their conversion to free radicals or to their effect in forming free radicals.

Inflammation — one of the commonest kinds of bodily disorder — is associated with free radical production, but the free radicals are probably the cause of the inflammation rather than the effect. However, the body actually uses free radicals to kill bacteria within the scavenging cells of the immune system — the *phagocytes* — and when excessive numbers of these are present in an inflamed area the free radical load almost certainly adds to the tissue damage, making everything worse. This is probably what happens in rheumatoid arthritis, for instance.

Free radicals also arise in the course of normal internal cellular function. This is called *metabolism* and it is, of course, essential. Metabolic processes require many chemical reactions that involve free radical action. The joining of chains of amino acids (*polymerization*) to form proteins, or the polymerization of glucose molecules into the polysaccharide glycogen, for instance, involve free radical action. In the course of metabolism important and potentially dangerous free radicals such as superoxide and hydroxyl radicals are produced. In most cases the process is automatically controlled and the number of free radicals does not become dangerously high. Fortunately, the body has, throughout the course of millions of years of evolution, become accustomed to coping with free radicals and has evolved various schemes for doing so.

Three Magical Enzymes

The breakthrough that caused medical scientists really to begin to look seriously at free radicals was the astonishing discovery that the body actually produces large quantities of a substance (an *enzyme*) whose only function is to break down the dangerous superoxide free radical. This enzyme is called *superoxide dismutase* (commonly called SOD by the scientists). There is no reason to be rude about this marvellous enzyme, for we really need it. This enzyme converts dangerous superoxide free radicals to the less dangerous hydrogen peroxide. This is still fairly powerful stuff, capable of turning us all blonde, and is quite damaging to tissues. Happily, the body produces another enzyme, called *catalase*, which immediately breaks down the hydrogen peroxide to water and oxygen, and all is well. There is a third natural antioxidant enzyme called *glutathione peroxidase* which also reduces hydrogen peroxide to water.

Each of these enzymes is made in cells under the instructions of a length of genetic code in DNA. Every cell in our bodies contains the instructions for making these three enzymes. So unless free radicals are important, why would evolution go to such lengths to protect the body against them?

That's something to think about.

2

Free Radicals and your Arteries

We don't give nearly enough thought and concern to our arteries. Many of us worry and complain about our joints, backs, lungs, legs, veins, skin, even our waterworks, but seldom, if ever, about our arteries. There are, of course, good reasons for this. One is that the effects of damaged arteries are mainly indirect. Another is that few of us really appreciate how fundamentally important they are. The truth is that artery trouble is far more serious than any of these other things we complain about.

The Menace of Atherosclerosis

By 'artery trouble' I mean one arterial disease, a very common condition called *atherosclerosis*. There are several other diseases of arteries but, apart from this one, all are comparatively rare. Atherosclerosis affects almost everyone — or, to be more accurate, almost everyone in the Western world. It begins in childhood and, in most cases, progresses very slowly throughout life. The degree to which it progresses matters a great deal and for a very simple reason: arteries carry blood; blood carries oxygen and vital nutrients. If these supplies are cut off, the various organs to which the blood is carried by the arteries will simply die.

14

If the blood supply is seriously restricted, they will suffer disorder or malfunction. Atherosclerosis causes narrowing or even blockage of the affected arteries. This means that less of the vital blood gets through to the organ or part. If the organ is the heart and the narrowing is excessive, the result is a heart attack, possibly death; if it is the brain, the result is a stroke; if it is a leg, the result is gangrene.

Atherosclerosis affects certain arteries more often than others and is particularly liable to occur in those supplying the heart, brain and the legs. But it can affect almost any arteries and can lead to dire consequences for the eyes, the kidneys, the intestines, some of the endocrine glands and other parts of the body. Atherosclerosis kills more people than any other single disease or cause. It also has a devastating effect on the quality of life of millions, crippling them with angina pectoris and agonizing leg pain on walking and, in other cases, causing progressive and distressing dementia.

Although we have known for years that there is a relationship between diet and atherosclerosis, it is only recently that it has become apparent that the actual damage to the artery that leads to the dangerous narrowing is caused by free radicals. This is why I have put it at the top of the list for consideration in a book on this subject.

What is Atherosclerosis?

The arteries are the tough, elastic, thick-walled tubes that carry blood, under fairly high pressure, from the heart to the various parts of the body. This blood is fresh from the lungs where it has picked up a good supply of oxygen, and it also carries the body fuel glucose from the liver and the intestines. Both oxygen and glucose are essential for life and health. The brain and the heart are especially sensitive to

15

lack of oxygen and glucose. If the supply of these vital substances is cut off for more than a few minutes death, or severe brain or heart damage, is inevitable. After the oxygen and glucose have been supplied to the tissues, the blood returns to the heart by way of the low-pressure, thin-walled veins to complete the circulation.

Atherosclerosis affects only arteries, not veins. It is a degenerative disease that starts in the first year of life with fatty streaks in the linings of the arteries. These are present in almost all Western world children and are believed to be the first stage in the process, although not necessarily the sites at which, much later in life, *plaques* will develop. Plaques are white or yellowish-white raised areas on the inner surface of the arteries, varying in size from about a third of a centimetre (one eighth of an inch) across to one and a half centimetres (just over half an inch) across. In severe cases the plaques are so numerous that they run together to form large masses. These plaques are made of an outer zone of mixed fibrous tissue, phagocyte cells and abnormal numbers of muscle cells with a core consisting of a disorganized mass of cell debris and fatty tissue, mainly cholesterol. Around the edges of the plaques are many tiny abnormal blood vessels that have budded out from the wall of the artery.

How Does Atherosclerosis Cause Harm?

The arteries most commonly and severely affected by atherosclerosis are the main arterial trunk of the body — the *aorta* — and its immediate branches. In particular, atherosclerosis affects the *coronary arteries*, the two branches of the aorta that supply the heart muscle with blood; the branches that run down to supply the legs; the *carotid* branches than run up the neck to supply the brain; and their branches that form a network under the brain. Although the branches to the kidneys and intestines are usually spared, it is common for the openings in the aorta for these branches to be severely narrowed by atherosclerosis.

Arteries are not usually closed off completely by plaques. What happens is that the surface of plaques becomes rough and sometimes broken down (ulcerated). This allows the blood to contact the underlying tissue. Blood is designed to clot whenever it comes in contact with body tissue other than blood vessel linings. So clotting on top of athcromatous plaques is very common. This is called *thrombosis* and, of course, such a clot can readily close off the artery altogether. Coronary artery thrombosis is the principal cause of heart attacks; cerebral artery thrombosis causes strokes, with all their frightening consequences of paralysis, speech and vision disturbance and general disablement. Even more serious strokes occur if small brain arteries are so damaged and weakened by atherosclerosis that they burst. The resulting bleeding around or into the brain is called *cerebral haemorrhage* and the effects are devastating.

Apart from the risk to the brain, heart and other organs, the damage to the aorta itself commonly leads to weakening of the wall and the pressure of the blood in this vessel is so high that the result is often a dangerous ballooning out of the aorta — a condition known as *aneurysm*. It is hardly necessary to state that an aortic aneurysm is a highly dangerous condition and that the consequences of bursting hardly bear thinking about.

So severe atherosclerosis is a condition to be avoided at all costs. Any knowledge about the ways in which it comes about is valuable knowledge, and any measures that could retard the progress of the disease would be priceless. That knowledge now exists and there is good reason to believe that we *do* have ways of limiting the worsening of this dreadful condition. Forget any ideas you may have that this is simply a matter of cutting down your intake of cholesterol. There is far more to it than that. Cholesterol is an essential body ingredient. Every cell contains cholesterol, and each day a large amount of cholesterol comes down your bile duct from your liver, where it is synthesized, and is reabsorbed into your blood. Certainly, a reduced intake of saturated fats will help, but there is always plenty of cholesterol in your body to be laid down in the atherosclerotic plaques, *if the process that leads to this dangerous deposition is operating.* Happily, we are now beginning to understand this process and we know that free radicals are deeply involved.

How Do Free Radicals Cause Atherosclerosis?

Cholesterol and other fatty materials (*lipids*) are transported around in the bloodstream in the form of tiny fatty bodies known as *lipoproteins*. These come in two main kinds, the low-density lipoproteins (LDLs) and the high-density lipoproteins (HDLs). The density comes from the proportion of protein present. HDLs have a lot of protein and a little cholesterol; LDLs have a lot of cholesterol and a little protein. LDLs carry cholesterol and other fats from the liver to the tissues — including the arteries — and HDLs carry cholesterol and fats from the tissues to the liver. LDLs can be thought of as the 'baddies' and HDLs as the 'goodies'.

Scientists have known about this for several years and have also known that if you eat a lot of saturated fats — stable fats with no double bonds between the carbon atoms, that are solid at room temperature — you will have lots of

LDLs in your blood. If you eat only polyunsaturated fats — fats with many double bonds, that are usually liquid at room temperature — you will have far fewer LDLs in your blood. What has not been known is how the cholesterol from the LDLs gets into the atheromatous plaques.

How Lipoproteins Become Dangerous

Lipoproteins are not, by themselves, much good at penetrating intact tissue. The way they work is to be taken to the site where their materials are required by blood vessels so tiny that the LDLs are able to get into direct contact with their target cells. Recent research indicates, however, that LDLs that have been attacked by free radicals and oxidized (see pp.9—10) are much more ferocious than normal tame LDLs. Oxidized LDLs can, apparently, fight their way through the inner lining layers of the walls of arteries so that they can deposit their loads under the surface layer. Some scientists have also proposed that free radicals also act in other ways — by injuring lining cells (*endothelium*) and smooth muscles cells in the vessel wall; by preventing scavenging cells (phagocytes) from doing their job; and by promoting the formation of the large phagocyte *foam cells* in which the cholesterol accumulates in the plaques. Significantly, research has shown that in rabbits with very high blood cholesterol levels, those given the antioxidant probucol — a drug related to BHT (see p.82) — develop fewer atherosclerotic plaques than those not given the drug. Probucol has also been used in humans.

So the present view on the production of atherosclerotic plaques is that LDLs do not, unless oxidized, help to form the plaques. Dr Hermann Esterbauer, of the University of Graz, Austria, a foremost researcher in the field of free radical damage to arteries, speaking at a conference at the

New York Academy of Sciences on the health implications of vitamin E, stated that there was strong evidence that free radical oxidation of LDLs was the essential fact and that unless LDLs were oxidized they were not capable of forming plaques. Delegates at the conference were told that the natural antioxidants in the LDLs were depleted by the free radicals to the point where they could no longer prevent damaging chain reactions caused by free radicals.

At the same conference, Dr K. Fred Gey of Hoffmann-LaRoche, Basel, and a Professor at the Institute of Biochemistry and Molecular Biology, University of Berne, reported the results of an interesting survey. This study, co-sponsored by the World Health Organization, was into the reasons for the striking differences in the mortality, in different countries, from heart disease caused by atherosclerosis of the coronary arteries. It had involved 11,000 men aged 40–59 from 12 countries. In some countries the death rates from heart disease was much higher than in others. Men living in Scotland and Finland, for instance, were four times as likely to die from heart disease than men living in Italy or Switzerland. There must clearly be some explanation for this remarkable difference, and Dr Gey suggested that it might have been found. In the course of the survey, the levels of antioxidants (vitamins E and A) in the blood of the subjects were monitored over a four-month period. The results were remarkably suggestive. In those with low levels of these vitamins the death rates were higher than in those with higher levels. This was not a marginal difference. Studies of previous risk factors, such as smoking, high blood pressure and high blood cholesterol, could predict an increased risk of heart disease with an accuracy of only 50 per cent. When the blood levels of these vitamins were also taken into account, the accuracy rose to 94 per cent.

It is probably worth mentioning, in this context, that —

as reported in the *Scottish Medical Journal* in 1989 — middle-aged Scottish men eat very little fruit and green vegetables. A pure coincidence?

3

How Free Radicals
Can Damage your Heart

In 1991 the prestigious weekly British medical magazine *The Lancet* carried a leading article — a report produced by the heart research unit in the Department of Cardiology and Medicine of the University of Edinburgh. This report, by Dr R. A. Riemersma and colleagues, described a research study into whether there was any connection between the levels of certain vitamins in the body and the risk of having angina pectoris. The vitamins concerned were vitamins C, E and A and the substance beta-carotene that is converted by the liver into vitamin A. There was more to this trial than immediately meets the eye.

About Angina

Angina pectoris is not, as is commonly thought, a disease, but a symptom. It is the often agonizing, tight, gripping, constricting pain 'like a steel band around the chest' that is felt by the sufferer after a certain, often predictable, amount of exertion. Angina usually comes on after walking for a particular distance, more quickly on a cold day or when walking against the wind, and especially when walking uphill. It may be brought on by anxiety or emotion. Sometimes the pain passes down the arms, especially the left arm; sometimes it radiates through to the back or up into the neck. Altogether a very unpleasant and worrying experience.

Angina is worrying because the trouble comes from the heart and is caused by asking the heart to work harder than it comfortably can with the limited oxygen and glucose supply available to it. This supply is limited because the arteries that carry the blood to the heart muscle — the coronary arteries — have been narrowed by atherosclerosis (see pp.14—18). Atherosclerosis is the disease; angina is the symptom. In the case of most affected people — usually men — the heart can beat away satisfactorily when the person is at rest. But during exertion, the heart has to work harder to pump additional blood to the muscles and there comes a point at which the narrowed coronary arteries cannot supply the needed increase in blood flow. When this happens, the heart complains. Waste materials accumulate around the heart muscle cells and these stimulate pain nerve endings. Many people with angina go on like this for years, but in some the condition gradually worsens until it may occur even at rest. In others the angina becomes more rapidly unstable and there is a serious risk that a coronary artery, or a large branch, may become completely blocked, causing coronary thrombosis — a heart attack.

Angina and Vitamins

Dr Riemersma's paper was especially interesting for several reasons. First, there is an obvious relationship between angina pectoris and the risk of heart disease: both are caused by the same arterial disorder — atherosclerosis. Second, the vitamins the report studied are antioxidants that attack free radicals. Perhaps most interestingly of all, the study — carried out by scientifically very well-informed people

— implied a presumption that there might well be a connection between free radicals and heart disease. The results of the study confirmed this presumption. No connection was found between vitamin A levels and angina. The results for vitamin C were confused by the fact that vitamin C levels are lower in smokers than in non-smokers, and since smoking is an established risk factor for heart disease this could not be attributed to low levels of the vitamin. But so far as vitamin E was concerned, there was no doubt about the result. Even after taking into account smoking, blood pressure, obesity and blood cholesterol levels, the fact were clear. Men with low blood levels of vitamin E were significantly more likely to have angina than men with higher levels.

The authors of the paper concluded that '. . . some populations with a high incidence of coronary heart disease should supplement their eating habits with more cereals, vitamin-E-rich oils, vegetables, and fruit'. The paper brought out some other very interesting points. As explained in Chapter 2, low-density lipoproteins (LDLs) altered by oxidation by free radicals are believed to be the main factors in the development of the plaques that narrow arteries in coronary artery disease. The authors of this paper draw attention to American research that showed that when vitamin E is added to cells grown in culture in the laboratory it blocks the oxidation changes in LDLs. They also point out that the protective polyunsaturated fats are very vulnerable to attack by free radicals, which can start a chain reaction causing them, in turn to become free radicals. This chain reaction can be prevented by vitamin E.

Although I have highlighted this paper, I would emphasize that this is but one of many hundreds of professional articles dealing with free radicals and heart disease that have been published in the medical press in recent years. Almost all of these support the view that free radicals have a highly significant part to play in causing heart disease.

Free Radicals and Heart Attacks

A heart attack is different from angina. It is the consequence of an actual blockage of a coronary artery or one of its branches. In some cases the heart attack is caused by a temporary spasm of a coronary artery so that it almost closes off for a time. The effects are the same. Heart attacks are not related to exertion, like angina, but can come on at any time. The pain is similar in nature but often more severe and it does not pass off on resting, but goes on and on. There is often a terrifying sense of impending death which, unfortunately, is often justified.

When a part of the heart muscle is completely deprived of its blood supply it becomes swollen and soon dies. This will weaken the heart's action and may sometimes weaken the wall of the heart, but is not necessarily fatal. With luck the dead patch of muscle forms a strong scar and the heart continues to beat satisfactorily, although it is capable of less powerful action than before. Sometimes this process is repeated several times, and with each attack the heart is damaged further. In such cases, heart failure — the inability to keep the blood circulating adequately — is likely to occur.

Modern research suggests that the most important effect of free radicals occurs not at the time of the blockage, but when the damaged tissue, especially that around the dead zone, is trying to recover by widening nearby blood vessels. This response is called *reperfusion* and it is during this period that more oxygen becomes available and the maximum danger from free radicals occurs. This fact was dramatically illustrated in a paper published in *The Lancet* in April 1993. Free radical research has now progressed to the stage at which evidence of the presence of free radicals can actually be obtained by analyzing a small sample of the blood emerging in a vein from the area concerned. Such blood is examined by a very advanced method known as *electron paramagnetic resonance spectroscopy*. Samples have to be stored at very low temperatures in liquid nitrogen until they can be examined.

The *Lancet* paper describes the case of a 61–year–old man who was treated in hospital two and a half hours after having a heart attack. A special kind of X-ray, called *angiography*, showed that one of his coronary arteries was blocked. A fine tube (catheter) with a small balloon at one end was passed into the affected artery, pushed along to the obstruction, and the balloon inflated. The artery was successfully opened up. So far, the matter was routine. This procedure of coronary artery balloon angioplasty is a day-to-day routine, too commonplace to be reported in a medical journal. What was different about this case was that, before passing the balloon catheter, a second, very narrow-bore, tube had been passed into the patient's heart so that the tip lay near the opening of the vein — the coronary sinus — that returns the coronary artery blood to the circulation. This allowed samples of the blood passing through the affected area to be taken throughout the procedure. These were immediately frozen to await spectroscopy.

Unfortunately, an hour later, the coronary artery closed again and the procedure had to be repeated. Again, samples of blood emerging from the affected area were obtained and processed. This time, the artery remained open long-term and all was well. When the blood samples were studied by electron paramagnetic resonance spectroscopy it was found that, in both episodes, each time the artery was opened up *a flood of free radicals poured out of the area*.

This was an important confirmation of the widely-held view that a great deal of the damage that occurs in the course of a heart attack is caused by free radicals that are released *during the recovery phase*, whether from the body's natural recovery response by opening up nearby blood vessels, or whether due to medical intervention. The experts currently believe that it is the increased availability of oxygen, at this point, that initiates the production of free radicals.

Later Free Radical Damage

However, it seems that the free radicals still haven't completed their deadly work. It has been known for many years that as soon as the heart muscle is damaged by loss of its blood supply, millions of scavenging white blood cells (phagocytes) move into the area to start cleaning it up so that healing and scar formation can proceed. What was not known until recently is that this *leucocyte infiltration*, as it is known in medical jargon, is also associated with a burst of free radical production. The reason for this is that phagocytes actually use free radicals in their cleaning-up operations (see p.11).

In the case described here, the monitoring of free radicals was continued and, sure enough, between 9 and 24 hours later there was a rise in the output of free radicals that went even higher than when the coronary artery was opened up on the first and second occasions. Such free radical production is probably necessary, but there is a real possibility that it is also responsible for further damage to the heart. Phagocyte free radical over-production has been investigated in several other diseases. Results suggest that the phagocytes may commonly overdo free radical production. There is increasing evidence that a substantial proportion of the damage done in these processes is the result of phagocyte-produced free radicals as distinct from the damage caused by the original agents.

Practical Implications and a Warning

Scientific medicine looks for explanations of disease processes before attempting to find cures. 'Try-it-and-see' methods — known as *empirical treatments* — are all very well and are certainly adopted if the evidence for their efficacy is strong enough. But until there is a demonstrable explanation of how they work, there is always a lingering doubt, and this doubt is sometimes later found to have been justified. Now that so much is known about the role of free radicals in the production of disease damage, the stage is set for attempts at intervention to try to minimize this damage. Such intervention must obviously take the form of an attack on the free radicals, either by the use of various antioxidants or by other means.

Medical interest in this possibility is now intense and many trials are being conducted. I must emphasize, however, that the basic problem in heart attacks is the narrowing and obstruction of the coronary arteries. Everything possible must be done, from the earliest stage, to minimize the risk of such narrowing or blockage. Since free radicals play an important role in causing the arterial disease that brings about this narrowing, we have one obvious line of approach. It would be totally wrong, however, on this account to deflect attention from the importance of the already established risk factors — smoking, obesity, high blood pressure, lack of exercise and a diet high in saturated fats. Free radicals are not the whole story and anyone who thinks that a regular daily dose of vitamin E and vitamin C confers a licence to continue the life of an over-eating, over-weight, cigarette-smoking, physically idle couch potato would be very foolish indeed.

Official Interest

Coronary heart disease commonly attacks men at the peak of their productive capacity and usefulness to society. Quite apart from the tragedy of death and blighted lives, the disease is of enormous economic importance. In September 1991 the British Ministry of Agriculture and Food set up a major research programme into free radicals and heart disease and the value of the antioxidants vitamin C, vitamin E and beta-carotene. With a budget of £1,650,000, this was one of the most intense investigations into free radicals and antioxidants ever mounted. Such a programme takes time and the eight projects are expected to take at least three years. Their findings are, of course, awaited with the greatest interest.

Do you think you should wait, or is there, perhaps, something you should be doing about it now?

4

Free Radicals and Cancer

Here we get into deep waters. Let me say at once that the significance of free radicals in relation to cancer is much less clear than in the case of arterial and heart disease, and that, sadly, there is simply no question of any sort of breakthrough having yet been achieved. Free radical and antioxidant studies are by no means in the forefront of cancer research, at least at the moment, and we still don't know whether they will ever be. Nevertheless, a substantial amount of research *is* going on to see just how significant free radicals are in relation to cancer.

Cancer is also a very complicated subject and any account of it in a book of this kind must necessarily be simplified. Even so, some of the basics of the subject must be covered if this chapter is to provide any worthwhile information. I'm afraid some of it will make rather gloomy reading.

What is Cancer?

The word 'cancer' is a convenient term, applicable to at least 200 different conditions. Cancer can involve any tissue or organ of the body, either as a primary change in that tissue or organ, or by invasion from elsewhere in the body. Some cancers are so minor that they can be cured by a needle prick and ten minutes of painless surgery. Others are so malignant that long before any signs appear, the disease may already be beyond remedy, so that it later resists every attempt at treatment. The common carcinoma of the bronchus, caused by cigarette smoking, is often of this type. There is, however, an important sense in which cancer is a single disease. All tumour cells, whatever their origin and type, share a common set of basic changes and follow a common pattern of abnormal behaviour. All cancer cells show very similar, or even identical, changes.

All human body tissues are composed of cells. Tissue cells operate as communities, and are restricted in their growth and reproduction by controlling factors. Normal tissue cells remain localized in their particular organs, growing and reproducing very slowly and just sufficiently to make up for accidental cell death. One factor responsible is known as *contact inhibition*. When cells are tightly packed together and unable to move, they reproduce slowly. If the cell density is reduced, cell movement occurs and this is associated with an increased rate of reproduction. Liver cells, for instance, normally grow very slowly, no faster than is necessary to make up for wear and tear. But if a piece of liver is removed, surrounding cells will multiply rapidly, regenerating liver tissue, until the deficiency is restored. In cancer, the restraints on reproduction are removed and cell replication is rapid and unchecked. Unlike normal cells, cancer cells also frequently move into tissue foreign to their type and place of origin.

Benign and Malignant Tumours

Not all tumours are cancers. There are two categories of tumours, and the different is important. *Benign tumours* are not cancers at all, just lumps of cells which, while still closely resembling the tissue from which they have arisen — muscle, nerve, fat, blood vessel and so on — have begun to reproduce and multiply more rapidly than normal. Benign tumours remain intact and grow by expansion only.

The features of *malignant tumours* are quite different. Malignant tumour cells do not remain in a well-defined, circumscribed lump, insulated from surrounding tissue. They are essentially invasive, and stretch out in columns which pass into nearby tissues, crossing anatomical barriers, spreading along surfaces, seeding off into blood and lymph vessels, and usually reproducing and growing at a much faster rate than normal cells. A cancer starting with one small group of cells has to divide many times before reaching a mass large enough to be detected. The smallest such detectable mass is of the order of 1 g. Cancers are usually fatal when the tumour mass has reached 500 g to 1 kg. This size is reached after only 7 to 10 further doublings of the 1 g mass.

Mutations and Cancer

Malignant tumours are collections of cells which have suffered a mutation (change) in their genetic material (DNA). Most major mutations are lethal: the affected cell dies and no further harm is done. Some mutations, however, cause cells to reproduce in a disorganized and uncontrolled manner, causing a cancer. All important cell functions, especially reproduction, are under the control of DNA. Damaged DNA does not, of course, necessarily cause a cell to become cancerous, but certain kinds of DNA change will disrupt normal gene regulation, activate certain tumour-producing genes known as *oncogenes* and, in this way, induce cancer. Any agency that can damage DNA is thus potentially capable of causing cancer, and we know of a number of things — radiation, certain chemicals and viruses — that can cause these changes. Radiation and dangerous chemicals do their harm by producing free radicals, so these are clearly implicated in the stage of chemical damage to DNA.

How Cancer Spreads

Cancers spread in two ways. They burrow into and invade adjacent tissues and structures, becoming incorporated into them and often destroying them. But they have another, and even more dangerous, way of spreading. When an invading cancer encounters a small blood vessel, it can grow through the wall until it reaches the bloodstream, and small collections of cancer cells can then be carried off by the fast-flowing blood to be deposited in another part of the body. This is called *metastasis* and is the major cause of death in cancer. By this means, cancer cells from the lung or colon or prostate gland can be transported to the brain or bones or liver, to set up a new focus and continue to grow and invade in the new site. In the absence of effective treatment, metastatic cancer is almost always fatal. Unfortunately, many people with cancers apparently confined to one site already have small inapparent metastases (*micrometastases*) in distant parts of the body. So even radical surgical removal of the primary tumour may not cure the cancer, which may appear in the new sites. It is for this reason that anticancer drugs, which have their effect wherever the cancer may be throughout the body, are often given in addition to surgery in cases in which such metastases are suspected.

Degrees of Malignancy

Cancers vary enormously in the speed with which they spread locally and, consequently, in the readiness with which they form new colonies elsewhere. This tendency is called *malignancy* and malignancy may be low or high. A tumour of low malignancy may take many months or even years to cause trouble and may not spread distantly for a very long time, if ever. Unfortunately, tumours of high malignancy will sometimes have spread widely before the victim has any idea that anything is wrong. A skilled pathologist can often tell, by examining a thin slice of cancer tissue under a microscope, whether it is of high or low malignancy. In tumours of low malignancy, the cells quite closely resemble the parent tissue and form themselves into aggregates which are not greatly different in structure from the normal tissue from which they arise. Very malignant cells, on the other hand, are 'primitive' simple cells with little or no capacity to form recognizable tissues. It is this simplicity which makes it easier for them to spread.

The Effects of Cancer

Cancers are, of course, destructive. Some become very large and cause local effects by their sheer physical bulk — by compressing or displacing important structures. They erode and damage organs and blood vessels, block tubes, destroy vital functional tissue, form abnormal connections between organs and body cavities, promote internal bleeding and the production of abnormal quantities of fluid, and allow access to infecting organisms.

In addition, cancers have general effects. These are caused by chemical substances, often proteins, released by the tumour cells and carried throughout the body by the bloodstream. Some of these substances resemble hormones and can have widespread and severe effects. Some tumours manufacture a wide range of these hormone-like substances. The small cell cancers of the lung, for instance, can produce hormones affecting the calcification of bone, the lining of the womb, the output of the adrenal glands leading to high blood pressure and other effects, and the function of the kidneys leading to inability to excrete enough water. Breast cancers and some lung and kidney tumours can produce hormones which raise the levels of blood calcium to dangerous degrees, causing vomiting, excessive urinary output and coma.

In addition to the hormone-like effects, tumours produce a variety of general effects, not all of which are fully understood. These include nausea, loss of appetite, anaemia, fever, skin rashes, weakness, abnormalities of taste sensation and severe and progressive loss of weight. The end result is often the severely debilitated state, with gross weight loss, known as *cachexia*, and this is often terminal. Cachexia may result from malnutrition from bowel obstruction or defective absorption of food or simply from the loss of appetite which is a common feature of widespread cancer. In addition, tumour cells have a greater demand for amino acids — the 'building bricks' of protein — than normal cells, and may use these up at the expense of the patient's muscles so that body wasting occurs. The cause of death in people with widespread cancer is usually a combination of several factors such as cachexia, infection, internal bleeding and compression of vital tissue — such as the brain — by a growing tumour mass. Actual destruction of essential structures is a less common cause of death.

Diet and Cancer

It is now generally accepted that the incidence of many of the cancers which afflict Western societies could be reduced by modifying our diet. Much of this evidence comes from observing differences in the number of cases of various cancers in populations with different eating habits. Western diets contain a staggeringly large number of different ingredients and to the basic foodstuffs is added a legion of additional substances — condiments, flavouring agents, flavour enhancers, sweeteners, preservatives, colouring agents, emulsifiers, solvents, antioxidants, stabilizers, bulking agents, antifoaming agents and others. All of these are, of course, tested for safety, but their very number, and the possibility that some might act on others with harmful effect, impose a major problem for the government agencies concerned.

At present, only a few substances known to be capable of causing cancer have been identified as possible dietary elements. Such substances are known as *carcinogens*. An example of these is *aflatoxin*, a poison produced by the common food contaminant mould *Aspergillus flavus*. Aspergillus grows readily on damp grains and nuts and is a common contaminant of peanuts. It is believed to cause many thousands of cases of primary liver cancer each year in countries in which food is stored in unsatisfactory conditions. Most cases occur in people whose livers have already been damaged by hepatitis B.

Other known cancer-causing substances include *nitrosamines*, produced by overcooking or smoking of animal protein, but not yet positively identified as a cause of cancer in man; *nitrates* and *nitrite* preservatives, which may form nitrosamines from dietary protein; salt fish, widely eaten in the Far East and believed to be related to the development of cancer of the back of the nose; bracken fern, which is known to cause cancer in animals, is popular in Japanese diets and is thought to be associated with cancer of the oesophagus. Less certain are the suggestions that stomach cancer is caused by highly spiced food, highly acidic foodstuffs such as pickles, nitrates in water and irritants such as the concentrated alcohol in spirits. None of these has been definitely proved.

We know, however, that a high fat diet can cause cancer in animals. The United States National Research Council, in their 1982 report *Diet, nutrition and cancer,* judged that the evidence linking dietary fat and cancer in humans was stronger than for any other dietary constituent. They recommended, on these grounds alone, that the public should reduce fat intake, both saturated and unsaturated. The evidence consists mainly of the strong link, in various countries, between the number of cases of cancer, especially of the breast and colon, and the consumption of fat. The number of cases has increased proportionately with an increase in the fat intake and has also increased in immigrants to countries with a higher fat intake than the countries of origin. Remember, however, that a high fat intake nearly always implies a low fibre intake and it is probable that the effect may be caused by low dietary fibre rather than high dietary fat. The evidence linking high-fibre diets and a low incidence of cancer and other bowel diseases is very strong and is generally accepted.

World-wide Research

It is good to be able to report that, apart from the huge amount of general cancer research in progress — which has already made substantial advances into our understanding of the subject — a great deal of research specifically into the question of free radicals and cancer is under way. At least 28 human trials, sponsored by the American National Cancer Institute, are in progress to discover the role of dietary factors, including vitamin E, in the development of cancer. In Britain, too, much research is in progress. The Imperial Cancer Research Fund, the Medical Research Council, the Dunn Nutrition Unit and the Department of Community Medicine at Cambridge University, among many other authorities are engaged in long-term studies, involving thousands of subjects, into the effects of dietary elements on the incidence of cancer. Monitoring includes the subjects' intake of vitamin C, E, A and beta-carotene. Huge similar projects are also under way in France, Germany, Spain, Italy, Denmark, Sweden, the Netherlands and Greece.

Free Radical Activity Markers

In the course of these studies, hundreds of thousands of samples of blood and urine are being taken and analyzed and, although it is impracticable on such a scale to detect the free radicals themselves, these samples are, among other things, examined for signs of free radical action. This is done by looking for markers of high levels of oxidation (see pp.9—10). These markers include the substances malonaldehyde, fat dienes (hydrocarbons with two double carbon-to-carbon bonds in the molecule), damaged protein thiols (sulphur-containing organic compounds), and the blood proteins, such as albumin, that take up free radicals. The greater the free radical activity, the higher the levels of these substances in the blood sample.

Another way of assessing free radical action, of special significance in the cancer context, is the degree of free radical damage to DNA. This, too, is being monitored by careful examination of the DNA in white blood cells in the samples. We know that free radicals can promote damaging chain reactions in DNA and that DNA damage can cause cancer. Examination of the DNA in white cells can show indications of severance of the double helix, appearing as regions in which there has been random rejoining. In smokers, DNA damage can be detected in cells from the lining of the air tubes, where lung cancer starts. These cells are constantly being coughed up and can be examined for the number of fragments of DNA lying free in them — an index of the amount of DNA damage by free radicals.

Preliminary Findings

Reports, to date, suggest that vitamins C and E and beta-carotene do offer protection against certain cancers, such as those of the lungs, oesophagus (gullet), stomach and large intestine. In particular, vitamin C is believed by some experts to be the body's major protective element against stomach cancer. This, if true, is especially important, because stomach cancer is one of the most dangerous and least easily detected kinds, and is often fatally advanced before it is diagnosed.

We are still a long way from fully understanding the role of free radicals in the development of cancer. We do not even know whether their contribution is major or minor. There are, however, some very suggestive points in the story and since many cancers are so frightful and antioxidants — vitamins C and E — so safe, it is perhaps not surprising that many of the researchers engaged in this work are, like the author of this book, taking their regular daily doses of these vitamins.

Are you asking yourself whether, maybe, you should be doing the same?

5

Do Free Radicals Accelerate Ageing?

Like most people, you probably think that the human life span is steadily increasing. In fact this is not so. There is no indication that the natural span of human life — about 100 years — is lengthening. What is happening is that people are living longer and getting near to, or reaching, the normal upper age limit. Life *expectancy* is increasing because medical and technological advances are enabling an increasing proportion of people to avoid death before reaching the full span. Today, in Western societies, for the first time in history, most people can look forward, with reasonable confidence, to growing old.

What Puts the Limit on our Life Span?

No one now believes that there is a single gene that controls ageing or that determines how long an individual will live. It is becoming clear, however, that many characteristic age changes are determined by a generic programme. Genes, although present, may or may not be expressed, and they may be expressed at different periods in life. The programme that determines whether or not genes actually have an effect can be enormously influenced by environmental factors. One of these factors is diet.

One central fact about ageing is the number of times our body cells can divide and so reproduce themselves, so that tissue damage from wear and tear may be repaired. This process of cell *replication* is going on all the time in our bodies at different rates in different cell types. Those in the reproductive organs and those subject to most wear and tear (such as those of the skin or the lining of the bowel) require the most frequent division.

Growing Cells in the Laboratory

It is possible to investigate, in the laboratory, the number of times cell replacement cycles can occur. It is not difficult to arrange suitable nutrition for cells, so that they can be made to survive and reproduce themselves outside the body. *Tissue cultures* of this type are now commonplace. One of the most famous of these, the HeLa culture, which was started many years ago from some cancer cells taken from a patient called Helen Lane, appears to be immortal and is now serving various useful purposes in hospital and research laboratories all over the world. So long as the conditions of nutrition are satisfied, the cell culture will continue to grow without limit.

But the cells of the HeLa culture, and of all other such artificial cultures, are abnormal and are incapable of the many important functions required of healthy cells within the body. They are all cancer cells and all they can do is grow and reproduce. Cancer cells do not show the characteristic changes in the expression of genes that occur over repeated generations of cell division in normal cells. This is why they are often immortal.

When *normal* cells are cultured, it is found that there is a definite limit to the number of times they can reproduce. This number has been repeatedly checked in different trials.

Cells called *fibroblasts* from a fetus or young baby will double in number between 40 and 60 times and the culture will then die. The average of 50 population doublings is remarkably constant. But if cells are taken from a middle-aged man and cultured, the number of doublings before the cells die will be reduced to about 25.

Trials have shown that the limiting factor is not the age of the culture but solely the number of times the cells reproduce. Even keeping the cells in suspended animation by freezing for several years does not alter this fact. They will just resume where they left off, undergo the immutable 50 or so doublings, then die. Cells from a wide range of human donors, of ages from birth to 90 years, show a steady average decrease in the number of times they reproduce before the culture dies. There is a rare disease called *progeria*, in which, at 10 years of age, the sufferer has all the physical appearances of a person of 70. Cells from such a person show only 2 to 10 doublings before the culture dies.

Shortening Chromosomes

The reason for this finite number of doublings became apparent recently when Dr Calvin Harley, a biochemist at McMaster University, Hamilton, Ontario, discovered that older cells had shorter chromosomes than younger cells. Loss of genetic material will kill off cells. To prevent loss of vital genetic material, the ends of chromosomes are made of unimportant 'junk' DNA that carries no genes and can, apparently, be lost without ill effect. These end segments are called *telomeres*. With each cell division, some of this junk DNA is shaved off. Eventually, the whole telomere is lost so that some of the true genetic material is exposed and removed. When this happens the affected cells become irretrievably damaged. When the telomeres are lost, chromosomes, being 'bare-ended', sometimes stick together at the ends, thus interfering with cell division. Cancer cells have very short telomeres but somehow manage to preserve them — possibly by means of an enzyme, known to exist, that can build up telomeres. Cells that can preserve their telomeres can go on dividing indefinitely, so long as suitable nutrition is provided.

This principle of 50 cell population doublings does seem to put a definite limit on our life expectancy. But I am not implying that, barring accidents or disease, we will all live until our cells just stop dividing. In fact, more than 100 different changes in the structure and function of cells have been noted to occur, long before they lose the ability to replicate. These changes, which increase progressively as the number of cell divisions is used up, progressively impair the cell's ability to perform its proper functions. It is these changes which produce all the well-known signs of old age and which result in the death of the individual, around the age of 100 years, long before the cells cease to divide.

Do We Want to Live Longer?

Considerable research has been directed to the study of these cell changes, in the hope of being able to arrest them and prolong life. But do we really want to live longer than the 'allotted span' — about 100 years?

Certainly, age changes being what they are at present, it is doubtful whether there would be much point in it. I have put the question to many elderly and old people, most of them in possession of all the important faculties, and the general opinion is against undue prolongation. That view may, of course, be a reflection of the psychological adjustments that temper our awareness of the approaching end of life with a capacity for calm acceptance. It may also reflect such a decline in physical power or bodily comfort that life is not thought worth living.

Conceivably, were it to prove possible to slow the rate of cell ageing, the outlook of every well-preserved person of 90 might come to resemble that of a contemporary man or woman in the prime of life. In many exceptional individuals, such as Linus Pauling, it does, even now. But, at the present stage of medical advance, and accepting the inevitable physical deterioration of age, we might do well to be contented with the present normal span, and think ourselves lucky if we reach it. No one would argue, however, over the merits of a long, healthy and active life, or about the importance of investigating the factors that shorten or damage the quality of life.

What is Ageing?

On this question there is no general agreement among the experts. In spite of a great deal of research and the development of a completely new biological discipline known as *gerontology*, there are still fundamental arguments. Some take the straightforward view that ageing is no more than the totality of all the unrepaired cellular and tissue damage suffered during life. Such accumulated damage is clearly an important element in ageing, but is not necessarily the whole story.

The evolutionary biologist George C. Williams of Michigan State University has put forward an ingenious theory of ageing. He pointed out that some genes do not start to operate to the disadvantage of the individual until well after middle age. Genes which are destructive later in life but have advantages earlier in life are passed on by people to their children before they, themselves, are affected by them. Such genes are thus not eliminated by natural selection. Nature is interested in the continuation of the species, not the continuation of the individual. A number of such genes have been identified. The biologist T. B. L. Kirkwood of the British Institute for Medical Research points out that, in an evolutionary and survival context, any species must share its energy between body maintenance and efficiency of reproduction. This implies less than full attention to bodily repair and inevitable deterioration and death.

Free Radicals and Ageing

In general terms, the free radical theory of ageing proposes that free radicals are more readily and plentifully formed in older people. We know that free radicals can damage any tissue in the body. The outer membranes of cells, which contain fatty material such as cholesterol, are especially susceptible to damage by fat peroxidation by free radicals. Such increased free radical production and damage might result from the cumulative effect of environmental influences, or from a reduction in the availability of body antioxidants, possibly from an age-related diminution in the activity of natural antioxidants.

We have seen how the arterial disease atherosclerosis has widespread and serious damaging effects. This disease obviously contributes importantly to the bodily changes characteristic of ageing. I have also outlined the close link between free radical oxidation of low-density lipoproteins and the development of atherosclerosis.

The third link between free radicals and ageing is their undoubted effect on DNA. Not all the DNA occurs in the chromosomes. All cells contain thousands of tiny energy-producing bodies known as *mitochondria* and these, too, contain a genome of DNA. Interestingly the mitochondrial

DNA comes in the non-nuclear part of the cell and so is derived from the egg, not the sperm. It is thus inherited only from the mother. Mitochondrial DNA is now known to be especially vulnerable to free radical damage, possibly because it is so concerned with oxidative chemical reactions. Any unrepaired free radical damage to this DNA would have a serious effect on the continued functioning of the cell. Scientists have estimated that oxygen free radicals are responsible for about 10,000 DNA base changes (mutations) every day. The great majority of these are automatically repaired, but even the most efficient repair mechanism is unlikely to pick up and correct every mutation.

The Role of Antioxidants

It has now been established that there is a positive and important link between diet and longevity. In many animal species, life span can be increased up to 50 per cent by suitable modification of the diet. Whether this enhancement is due to a reduction in free radical action so that bodily antioxidants can more readily cope remains to be seen. There is evidence that rats on low-calorie diets suffer less free radical damage to their body proteins — the essential building materials of the body — than those on unrestricted diets. This may be because they have larger quantities of the important enzymes that protect against free radicals (see pp.12–13). Antioxidants are unlikely to be the whole story, for in rats living longer on restricted diets there is known to be increased expression of certain genes in liver tissue. So genetic factors are also probably involved.

There is, however, some more direct evidence of increased free radical action with age. Scientists at the University of Kentucky have been studying the performance of gerbils in running mazes. Old gerbils, on average, make twice as many mistakes as young gerbils. But if old gerbils are given the free radical-trapping antioxidant butyl-alpha-phenyl-nitrone (PBN) for two weeks, their performance improves so as to be every bit as good as that of young gerbils. When the PBN was stopped, they went back to making as many mistakes as before.

Proteins that have been damaged by free radical oxidation can be detected by highly sensitive tests for bits of amino acids (carbonyl groups) that are released in the course of the damage. Post-mortem examinations on human brains have shown more of these groups in old people than in those of young people. The probability is that antioxidants can make up for progressive, age-related deficiencies of the natural antioxidants that mop up free radicals in younger people.

The researcher Thomas Johnson of the University of Colorado has been able to breed a strain of roundworm with a life span more than twice that of others of the same species. The remarkable thing about these long-living worms is that they have significantly higher levels of the enzymes superoxide dismutase and catalase (see p.12) than their less fortunate friends. These enzymes are natural antioxidants and are exactly the same as those that protect humans against free radicals.

As long ago as 1956, the research scientist D. Harmon, writing in the *Journal of Gerontology*, suggested that free radicals are probably involved in the ageing process. Since then the free radical theory of ageing has become widely accepted. Gerontologists now generally believe that free radical damage to tissues is a central factor in the development of most of the age-related diseases — atherosclerosis, arthritis, loss of muscle and heart efficiency, arthritis, cataract, rheumatoid arthritis, lung disorders, skin deterioration and probably cancer.

Earl R. Stadtman, chief of the biochemistry laboratory at

the National Heart, Lung, and Blood Institute, National Institutes of Health, Bethesda, Maryland, writing in *Science*, the American general scientific journal, in August 1992, summarized the current scientific views on free radical oxidation of proteins and ageing. He confirmed the general opinion that free radicals are responsible for much damage to cell membranes and DNA, and described in detail the way proteins are attacked by hydroxyl radicals (see pp.6, 8), produced by radiation and ozone, and by hydroxyl and other radicals produced in the body. The evidence he quotes suggests that anything up to 50 per cent of the cellular protein in old people might be present in the damaged, oxidized form.

This very hard-headed scientist ends the paper with the carefully restrained statement: '. . . there is reason for hope that a pharmacological intervention may be found to ameliorate age-related disorders.' In other words, we have reason to believe that it may become possible to prevent the signs of ageing by taking antioxidant vitamins.

What do you think?

6

Free Radicals and your Eyes

As the medical literature on free radicals and antioxidants grows, an increasing number of body systems and medical conditions are shown to be affected. Although, so far, the visual system has received comparatively little attention, interest is growing and it seems probable that, before long, many eye disorders will be seen to be mediated by free radical damage. One major eye disorder, which affects millions of people and causes great distress, has, however, prompted a number of very interesting and productive research projects. That condition is cataract.

Cataract

Cataract has nothing to do with the outer lens of the eye — the cornea — nor is it, as is commonly believed, a 'skin' growing over any part of the eye. It is simply loss of transparency of the internal focusing lens of the eye — the 'crystalline' lens that lies immediately behind the coloured iris and that can be seen only through the pupil. The name arose centuries ago from the fanciful idea that the whiteness in the pupil — which is seen only in long-neglected cases — was a kind of waterfall descending from the brain. In a dense cataract the pupil may indeed appear white, but the appearance is due to a 'denaturing' of the delicate protein fibres within the lens, in a manner similar to the changes occurring in the white of an egg when it is boiled.

Even the most dense cataract never entirely eliminates perception of light so, although cataract can fog out any useful image, it never causes complete blindness in the sense that nothing is seen at all. An eye that can perceive no light at all has something more seriously wrong with it than simply cataract. Often the opacity involves only the rear part of the lens and so a person may have a severe defect of vision while still having a normal-looking eye.

Causes of Cataract

Although cataracts can be brought about by virus infection before birth, penetrating or blunt injury, severe diabetes, Down's syndrome and various other causes, the great majority of cataracts simply occur, apparently spontaneously, in elderly people. Most people over about 75 have some detectable loss of visual clarity from cataract. Many have a marked degree of visual deterioration, but because the effects of old-age cataract on vision come on so gradually, and adaptation is so good, a great many people with quite severe opacities will deny that there is anything wrong.

Eventually, however, many find that they cannot read or even watch TV with any satisfaction. Unfortunately, many people in this situation accept their disability as a 'normal' feature of ageing and do nothing about it. This is a great pity, as the results of cataract surgery, with intraocular lens implantation — assuming there is nothing else wrong with the eye — are excellent, and cataract operations are among the most successful of all surgical procedures. Indeed, the condition is so remediable that ophthalmic surgeons faced with patients suffering from severe loss of vision are usually mentally hoping that the trouble is cataract. In spite of this, the prospect of surgery on the eyes is usually daunting, sometimes terrifying, to the patient.

Symptoms of Cataract

Cataract cannot cause pain and never does. Its only effect is on the quality of vision. The condition comes on almost imperceptibly and nearly always progresses very slowly. Usually the progress of the opacification is steady, but sometimes there are brief accelerations and then longer periods when little change is apparent. Many cataracts alter the way in which different light wavelengths pass through the lens, so that red and yellow light can pass through more easily than blue light. Again, the effect is gradual and may not be readily noticeable, but after cataract surgery it is commonplace for patients to exclaim with pleasure at the unaccustomed colour of the sky or of blue objects.

Another effect of increased density in the lens is an increase in its power of bending light rays. This is known as an increase in the *refractive index* of the lens. The effect is that the person affected may become gradually more and more short-sighted. This often allows them, at least for a time, to read without reading glasses, and may even promote the illusion that the vision is improving. The ability to make out near detail is, however, always accompanied by blurring of distant objects. People in this situation sometimes buy a succession of ever-stronger glasses for distance vision and spend a lot of money in an eventually hopeless quest for visual clarity. There is no harm in this, except to the bank balance.

The most important symptom of cataract is progressive loss of visual clarity in the centre of the field of vision. This is very annoying and disabling, especially if the lens opacities cause scattering of the light. Some people first become aware that something is wrong when they find they have to give up driving at night because of the dangerously blinding glare from the headlights of approaching cars. Many, on the other hand, are quite unaware of such effects and simply recognize that they can't see so well as they used to.

Once the lens protein has become denatured and the fibres disorganized, there is no possible way to restore transparency. The only remedy is to remove the opaque lens completely and replace it with a tiny, optically perfect plastic lens implant of a power calculated to focus the eye correctly.

Cataract and Free Radicals

The mechanisms of the development of age-related cataract are still a matter of argument, but it is becoming increasingly obvious that oxidation of the lens protein is an important factor. The fine protein fibres of which the internal lenses are made are themselves transparent. The transparency of the lens as a whole depends on the uniformity of diameter of these fibres and the evenness and parallelity with which they are laid down in the lens. When protein is damaged, this uniformity of structure is lost, and the fibres, instead of transmitting light evenly, cause it to be irregularly refracted and even reflected. The result is severely defective vision.

The view that age-related cataract may be due to free radical damage is indirect but very strong and is based largely on the differences between the levels of antioxidants in the bodies of people with cataract compared with those in comparable people with clear lenses. These trials have been reported in various respectable medical and scientific journals such as the *British Medical Journal*, *Archives of Ophthalmology*, *Annals of the New York Academy of Science* and the *American Journal of Clinical Nutrition.*

One of the most impressive studies was carried out in the Department of Biomedical Sciences, University of Tampere, Finland, and published in the *British Medical Journal* in December 1992. In this project 47 people with cataract and a carefully selected comparable group of 94 people with clear lenses were compared. The normal 'controls' were selected to be as similar as possible to those with cataracts in terms of age, sex, occupation, smoking history, blood cholesterol levels, body weight, blood pressure and the presence or absence of diabetes. All had blood samples taken that were analysed by highly sensitive methods for levels of vitamin E and beta-carotene.

The results showed that there was a significant relationship between the levels of vitamin E and beta-carotene and the likelihood of having cataract. Low blood levels of these antioxidant vitamins were found in the cataract group; higher levels in the clear lens controls. People low in both vitamins were two and a half times as likely to have cataracts as those with higher levels. The authors of the study concluded:

Low serum concentrations of the antioxidant vitamins alpha-tocopherol (vitamin E) and beta-carotene are risk factors for end stage senile cataract. Controlled trials of the role of antioxidant vitamins in cataract prevention are therefore warranted.

Another study, carried out in Canada and reported at an international conference, involved 175 cataract patients and the same number of people with clear lenses. Again, this study showed a meaningful difference in the intake of vitamins E and C in the two groups. Those who had taken extra C and E vitamins for five years or more were significantly more numerous in the clear lens group than in the cataract group. The epidemiologist Professor James Robertson, head of the project, said: 'Supplementary vitamins C and E are associated with a significant reduction in risk of cataracts.'

Free Radicals and Ultraviolet Light

Many scientists now suspect that at least one source of cataract-producing free radicals is ultraviolet light — which is present in large quantity in sunlight. Some have even suggested that this is the reason why cataracts occur much earlier in countries such as India than in more temperate areas. It is already well established that ultraviolet radiation produces free radicals in tissue. Ultraviolet light is the cause of sunburning and of the age-related damage to skin found in people with a history of long exposure to sunlight (see pp.68—9). These are free radical effects. It is also the cause of much external eye irritation and of the condition of *pterygium* in which a fold of the membrane covering the white of the eye (the conjunctiva) moves across over the cornea. Surface eye tissues, being transparent, are very susceptible to ultraviolet light, and, in view of recent developments, it seems almost certain that these changes are induced by free radicals.

Because the internal lens of the eye is protected by the cornea and by a layer of water behind the cornea, both of which partially absorb ultraviolet light, ophthalmologists have been less ready to accept that ultraviolet light is an important cause of cataract. In recent years, however, this view has gained increasing support. The idea that free radicals are involved is supported by research conducted at the University of Maryland by biochemistry Professor Shambu Varma. Isolated lenses exposed to strong light stresses became cloudy, but this could be prevented if the solution in which the lenses were placed contained antioxidants. Professor Varma also recommended that people should take supplementary vitamins C and E, at least from around the age of 40, to protect the lenses against later cataract formation.

Free Radicals and the Premature Eye

Very small babies must often be nursed in atmospheres of oxygen in incubators if their lives are to be preserved. Unfortunately, all eye specialists have become familiar with the devastating effects of excessive oxygen on the eyes of these premature infants. Too much oxygen produces free radicals, and the immature tissues of the infants are especially vulnerable to their damaging effects. There is severe damage to the retina and an abnormal budding-out of fronds and tangles of new blood vessels that produce a white mass behind the lens, known as *retrolental fibroplasia*, which can completely obscure vision. Detachment of the retina may also occur, as may high degrees of short sight.

These tragic results have been seen only too often in the past in very small babies who have had to be incubated. Happily, now that doctors are alive to the risk and are carefully monitoring the amount of oxygen given, severe cases are much less common. Today, the effects are usually limited to scarring and distortion of the retinas and, of course, they vary widely. In one study of 572 infants of birth weight below 1,700 grams, half had visible signs of the disorder. Happily, the great majority of these cleared up without treatment. As might be expected, the lower the birth weight and the shorter the pregnancy, the greater the severity. Paediatricians often have to make agonizing decisions in which they must balance the risk to the life of the baby against the risk to its vision.

The premature eye is vulnerable because it already has a plentiful oxygen supply and an unusually high rate of oxidation. It also has a much higher than average number of mitochondria (see pp.45—6). Newborn babies have reduced blood levels of vitamin E. This typically rises to normal within two or three weeks, but in the case of premature infants this takes much longer. Such babies, therefore, have less antioxidant protection than they need.

It has, therefore, been very tempting to treat premature babies with vitamin E supplements. Here, great caution is needed. Not all free radicals are antagonistic to the body. Free radicals are the means by which certain of the cells of the immune system kill bacteria and viruses. It is comparatively easy in very small babies to reach very high levels of vitamin E in the blood and this may interfere with the necessary action against germs. The normal adult blood concentration of vitamin E is about 0.8 mg in every 100 cubic centimetre (100 millilitre). Some babies treated with vitamin E have had concentrations of as high as 5 mg per 100 cc, and an increased incidence of a serious bowel infection occurred in babies on such dosage. For this reason, although some trials have shown a significant decrease in free radical eye problems, the use of vitamin E in premature infants remains highly controversial.

What this work does indicate, however, is that vitamin E is a powerful substance that can have major effects in the body and that it should be treated with respect. People often operate on the principle that you can't have too much of a good thing. This principle certainly does not apply in the context of self-treatment with some of the vitamins. There is no reason to suppose that reasonable doses of vitamin E are likely to cause any harm to children and adults. Excess vitamin A and D can certainly be harmful (see pp.84, 92). Vitamin C appears to be remarkably safe.

The evidence for the protective value of vitamin C and

E against cataract is very persuasive. Maybe this is yet another good reason to consider taking them, especially if you have reached the prime of life.

7

Do You Inhale Free Radicals?

Smoking is by far the most dangerous use of addictive substances, and, in spite of an enormous amount of advice and pressure, unhappily remains one of the major health issues of today. For every lung cancer death caused by smoking, there are three deaths from other smoking-related diseases. Smoking is expected to cause 2,100,000 deaths in 1995 in the developed countries alone. During the 1990s smoking will cause about 30 per cent of all deaths in the 35 to 70 age group, making it the largest single cause of premature death. Although large numbers of people have now been able to give up, and smoking has become, in more than one sense, a divisive social issue, there are still many who seem unable to conquer this addiction. Recent research into the relationship between free radicals and the damaging effect of smoking may, I hope, provide some smokers with better motivation to stop this hazardous practice.

Why Do People Smoke?

This is a question smokers often ask themselves and usually have difficulty in answering. There are obviously some advantages, but they do not seem particularly compelling. There is pleasure in observing the geometric perfection of a fresh cigarette. There is a basic satisfaction, known as *oral gratification*, in putting things into one's mouth. There is the slight lift of the spirits experienced within 10 seconds of the first drag, and the relief of the sense of tension which has prompted the person to smoke. There is the acquired pleasure in the taste of the smoke. Many people enjoy offering cigarettes to their friends. Some people don't know what to do with their hands in company and find cigarettes solve this problem. These are the reasons for which people act so gravely against their own interests, waste money, give themselves bad breath, body odour and stained fingers, and systematically damage many of the systems of their bodies so that, even if the worst does not happen, their long-term quality of life is likely to be substantially reduced.

Why Don't People Stop?

Today everyone knows that cigarette smoking is dangerous and damaging, and yet millions continue to smoke. What is it that prevents so many people from giving it up? The truth is that it is always easy to find reasons or excuses for continuing to do what we want to do. This is called *rationalization* and we all regularly use this convenient psychological mechanism. Rationalizations about smoking include that it is a drug addiction and so impossible to break; that the doctors don't really know what they are talking about; that the evidence about cancer is all statistical, and thus suspect; that grandfather smoked all his life, and lived to be 90, hale and hearty; and so on. Rationalizations have nothing to do with logic, although they often possess a kind of pseudo-logic.

People smoke because the impulse to self-gratification is powerful, central and natural. We have to recognize this and admit that the impulse is one of our major motivating forces. One might hope that the yielding to this impulse should be under the control of the reason, and that we should be able to identify and avoid acts of immediate, short-term gratification that are likely to have ungratifying effects in the long term. Apparently not. Even the most intelligent of us regularly succumb to the desire for self-gratification, while knowing that the activity indulged in may be seriously harmful.

Why Smokers Continue

Most smokers want to give up but find great difficulty in doing so. There are many reasons for this. Cigarettes are cheap and very easily obtained. They are portable and of a consistent quality. They present no danger of overdosage. They do not produce intoxication, slurred speech, staggering gait. There is almost no occasion that cannot be made an occasion for a smoke, and many occasions have become linked with smoking, as an automatic conditioned reflex. People smoke after a meal, after sexual intercourse, before any important occasion, after any important occasion, and so on. If anxious, a cigarette can calm; if depressed, a cigarette can give a lift.

Another reason for people continuing to smoke is that their motives for stopping are usually ineffective. Smokers really don't take seriously the statistics about the risks of lung cancer. This is probably because the figures convey nothing of the real horror of this terrible disease, and because of the ease with which we can refuse to believe something that threatens our comfort. Emotional reasons don't work; neither do logical reasons. Even so, I believe logical reasons are better than emotional reasons and, in the hope that an explanation of the way in which smoking damages the body may provide such a logical reason,

I would urge smokers, or the friends and relatives of smokers, to read on.

Free Radicals and Smoking

Cigarette smoke contains a very nasty mix of free radicals, and some of the thousands of substances present in inhaled smoke and absorbed into the body during smoking can also produce free radicals. Free radicals bring about many, if not most, of the serious bodily effects associated with smoking, especially the damaging effects on the arteries. Dr Hermann Esterbauer, of the University of Graz, Austria, a prominent researcher into the biological effects of free radicals, points out that smoking, a long-recognized risk factor for heart attacks, leads to low-density lipoprotein (LDL) free radical oxidation, probably from extra radicals produced in the body by absorbed smoke ingredients.

There is also growing speculation that the cancer risk in smoking may be largely due to free radicals. This speculation is based on some quite strong evidence. As we have seen, although free radicals are hard to detect directly, there are various indirect ways of determining that they have been busy. Protein breakdown products of oxidation can be detected and so can indicators of DNA oxidation damage. When DNA is damaged, it immediately tries to repair itself. This repair work is done by enzymes called *exonucleases*. When these enzymes get to work they release a compound called 8-hydroxydeoxyguanosine. This gets into the blood and is excreted in the urine.

In the December 1992 issue of the scientific cancer journal *Carcinogenesis* there is a paper from research scientists at the University of Copenhagen, Århus University and the Danish Cancer Registry. This paper reports the results of a trial in which the quantities of this tell-tale compound in the urine of smokers was compared with the quantities in non-smokers' urine. The figures speak for themselves. The smokers' urine contained 50 per cent more 8-hydroxydeoxyguanosine than that of non-smokers. This means that smokers' DNA is suffering a considerably greater rate of damage compared with non-smokers.

This additional damage could be coming either from the free radicals present in cigarette smoke or from free radicals produced in the body. We know that smokers have a higher metabolic rate (the rate of build-up and break-down of body biochemicals) than non-smokers — typically 10 per cent to 15 per cent higher. Raised metabolic rate accelerates all kinds of biochemical reaction pathways and some of these produce free radicals.

It would be quite wrong to leave you with the impression that researchers believe that free radicals are the most important cause of smoking-induced cancer. There is plenty of evidence that other mechanisms are also at work, especially the effects of the binding to DNA of certain aromatic hydrocarbons found in cigarette smoke. Nevertheless, the current interest in the role of free radicals in this context is intense.

Antioxidants and the Risk of Cancer

The tell-tale indicator of DNA damage in the urine of smokers makes them particularly suitable subjects for investigating whether antioxidants such as vitamin C, vitamin E and beta-carotene can reduce the risk of cancer. Many workers in the field now believe that the time has come for long-term trials of antioxidants. There are, however, difficulties. People who know what smoking can do to the human body have ethical qualms about any advance that may encourage smokers to continue. The scientists concerned are, however, at pains to point out that work of this kind is *not* undertaken in the hope of trying to make smoking safer, and some preliminary work has been done.

In addition to the monitoring of urine for 8-hydroxydeoxyguanosine, there are other ways of detecting rates of free radical damage to DNA. Lung cancer is not really cancer of the lung substance itself but of the lining (the *epithelium*) of the air tubes (*bronchioles*) in the lungs. Bronchial carcinoma — the medical term for lung cancer — starts in this epithelium. Researchers are, therefore, extremely interested in the epithelial cells that are present in coughed-up sputum. When cell division is defective — an early feature of a change in the direction of cancer — short lengths of DNA are left in the fluid within the epithelial cells. These fragments are called *micronuclei* and the proportion of them is, of course, of great significance.

In a paper in the *British Journal of Cancer* at the end of 1992, the researcher Geert van Poppel and colleagues describe how the proportion of micronuclei in epithelial cells coughed up by smokers can be reduced by 30 per cent by taking large doses of the antioxidant beta-carotene.

This result, although of the greatest scientific interest, has alarmed some of the scientists concerned with this problem. The epidemiologist Professor Richard Peto FRS, of the Imperial Cancer Research Fund in Oxford, is worried that news about the value of antioxidants may lead smokers to believe that they can safely continue so long as they take their vitamins. He points out that it is still too early to say that DNA damage by free radicals is the most important reason for the high incidence of cancer in smokers.

Whether it proves to be so or not, smoking will remain one of the most dangerous of human activities.

Smoking and Genetic Disorders

Epidemiologists at the University of North Carolina have recently carried out an important study of 15,000 children born between 1959 and 1966. This showed that the children of men who, prior to the birth, had smoked more than 20 cigarettes a day were twice as likely to suffer from certain genetic defects such as cleft lip and palate and congenital heart disorders. Another associated study by scientists at the National Institute of Environmental Health at North Carolina found that leukaemia and lymph node cancer were twice as common in the children of male smokers as in the children of non-smokers. Brain tumours were also significantly more common. Interestingly, the effect seems to be on sperm DNA but not on egg (ovum) DNA. No genetic links have been found that can be attributed to smoking by the mother. This is probably because cells forming sperms are far more often in a state of division (mitosis) than are eggs. Mutations occur mostly during mitosis because repair activity is temporarily halted during this phase.

Reporting these findings at an international conference on environmental causes of cancer in February 1993, the American biochemist Bruce Ames, of the University of California at Berkeley, said: 'I am already convinced that a good proportion of the birth defects and child cancers are coming from male smokers.' Ames pointed out that much of the damage resulting from smoking comes from strongly oxidizing compounds in cigarette smoke, such as free radicals.

When such oxidation damage affects the general body cells, the injury is limited to the person concerned. The worst that can happen is that the person dies of cancer. But if free radicals damage the DNA in the cells that produce sperms, then some of the sperms will carry mutant DNA.

If a child happens to be produced by fertilization by such a damaged sperm, congenital defects will result and the resulting mutations can, as Ames put it, cause 'an effect that will reverberate down the generations'.

Ames points out that because there is about eight times as much vitamin C in seminal fluid as there is in blood, this antioxidant vitamin *must* play an important role in protecting sperms from genetic damage. Since, like all cells in the body, sperms are attacked by about 10,000 oxidizing reactions every day, they clearly need such protection. The amount of vitamin C in the diet is sensitively reflected in the amount present in the seminal fluid. Even more significant, a low dietary intake of vitamin C immediately produces a substantial increase in the amount of 8-hydroxydeoxyguanosine (see above). This means that more DNA is being damaged. The current official recommended daily allowance of about 60 mg is too low to produce enough vitamin C in semen to reduce this DNA damage to safe levels. Research suggests that a minimum daily intake of 250 mg should suffice. Smoking uses up much of the vitamin C levels in the body to cope with the large amounts of oxidizing compounds in absorbed smoke, so smokers are clearly at greater risk.

The British Ministry of Agriculture, Fisheries and Food has been interested in free radicals and smoking for some time, and a project has been running since 1992 to compare blood antioxidant levels (see pp.66, 82—3) in smokers and non-smokers. One of the scientists involved in this project, Gary Duthie, explained that every time a smoker takes a puff at a cigarette, he or she takes in a huge dose of free radicals. The number has been estimated at around one hundred million million per inhalation. This project will also test the theory that supplementary doses of vitamin C, vitamin E and beta-carotene can reduce the amount of cell damage caused by free radicals.

Smoking and Cataract

If you are especially interested in cataract you will already have read the chapter on free radicals and your eyes, in which are outlined the nature and effects of this disabling but readily remediable condition. There is, however, a recently discovered and important link between cataract and smoking — a link that should be of interest to everyone.

Separate studies for men and women on smoking and the incidence of cataract, published in the *Journal of the American Medical Association* in August 1992, have shown that people who smoke 20 or more cigarettes a day are about twice as likely to develop cataract as non-smokers. The men concerned were 22,071 American doctors and the women were 50,828 American registered nurses. The explanation of the incidence of cataract has to be related to the lower concentrations of the antioxidant vitamins C, E and beta-carotene in the blood of smokers. Lens damage in cataract is oxidative damage of the lens protein. Cigarette smoke is rich in free radicals and other oxidative substances such as aldehydes. We know that free radicals from cigarette smoke can damage proteins. In view of all this it is hardly surprising that smokers are more prone to cataract than non-smokers.

A Warning

There is much in this chapter to encourage the idea that smoking can be made safer by taking vitamins. As we have seen, smokers are very good at latching on to any convenient rationalization. This one would be particularly dangerous. In my professional experience I have seen far too many tragedies, far too many promising lives cut short, far too many people turned into respiratory and cardiac cripples to be able to contemplate smoking with equanimity. We are now beginning to understand in much more detail how smoking damages the body and this understanding includes details of a great many processes that have nothing to do with free radicals.

Take the advice of a former smoker who, 30 years ago, was lucky enough to discover the facts in time — give it up.

8

Other Free Radical Effects

This chapter is a bit of a rag-bag as it deals with a number of seemingly unconnected conditions. But there is a common theme as these are all conditions in which free radicals have been found to play an important part. One of these conditions — skin ageing — is of special interest, as it is one of the first of what I hope will be a long list of conditions in which it has been shown possible to reverse, at least to a degree, free radical damage. This chapter also covers some little-known facts about the scavenging cells of the body — the phagocytes — and takes a brief glimpse at the intriguing theory that red wine may be good for you.

Skin Ageing and Free Radicals

Doctors have known for years that sunlight is damaging to skin. This was not a particularly clever deduction as the evidence has been around for centuries. A direct comparison of the skins of white people living cloistered lives with those of people who spend their days in the open, especially in tropical and sub-tropical areas, shows that, while the former remain smooth and elastic, the latter become wrinkled, discoloured and lax. Many sun-loving people of European or American origin who live for years in hot areas suffer devastating skin damage, with drooping, sagging folds, extensive fine wrinkling, and a much higher than average incidence of the three common skin cancer: rodent ulcer (basal cell carcinoma), squamous cancer (squamous epithelioma) and malignant melanoma.

Scientists have known for decades that this damage is caused by radiation — specifically ultraviolet radiation from the sun. The most obvious effect of this radiation is on the elastic collagen protein of the skin which becomes reduced in quantity and altered in quality. Loss of support to the small blood vessels leads to their expansion and prominence, as 'broken veins' (telangiectasis). Skin specialists, recognizing that these changes are the result of light damage over long periods, call them *photo-ageing*.

Tretinoin and Ageing Skin

The new knowledge concerns the way that ultraviolet radiation actually causes the damage. Paradoxically, in this case, the treatment came before the explanation. In 1986 a paper appeared in the *Journal of the American Academy of Dermatology* entitled 'Topical tretinoin for photo-aged skin'. This paper recounted how the ratio of sun-damaged to normal skin collagen could be markedly reduced by treatment with tretinoin. This was followed by similar papers in other journals, including one in the *Journal of the American Medical Association* entitled 'At last, a medical treatment for skin ageing'. Some trials involved large numbers of patients treated with tretinoin over a period of several months. Tretinoin is *all-trans-retinoic acid* and is the active form of vitamin A in all the tissues of the body except the retina. It is a powerful antioxidant. Taking tretinoin is not the same as taking vitamin A.

We now know, of course, that the ultraviolet light causes production of free radicals and that it is these that do the damage. By the time this became clear, dermatologists already knew that they could partially reverse the effects of solar radiation on the skin by using tretinoin. In a typical trial of this treatment, one side of the face of volunteers was treated with 0.05 per cent tretinoin cream once a day and the other side treated with the cream base without the tretinoin. At the end of 12 weeks, skin thickness, as measured by ultrasound and other methods, had increased by 10 per cent.

Other trials over longer periods of treatment showed improvement in skin thickness, in the roughness of the skin and in fine wrinkling, but, as might be expected since much damage had already been done, no change in sagging, age freckles (lentigines) or broken veins. Thickening of the outer skin layer, the *epidermis*, was, in many cases, remarkable, and could be as great as two and three-quarter times. Almost all the people in the trial suffered some degree of minor inflammation with itching and a feeling of tightness, a side effect, but this settled on stopping the cream applications for a day or two and the treatment could then be safely resumed.

These trials make it clear that people whose skin has already been severely damaged by the sun are likely to derive much less benefit from tretinoin treatment than people who have had less exposure to solar radiation. Tretinoin, under the trade name of *Accutane*, is also widely used in the treatment of the adolescent skin disease acne, in which it is highly effective. It has been used mostly in the USA, but also widely in Britain. It was introduced in 1982 and has been used by over a million people world-wide.

Risk from Tretinoin

The manufacturers repeatedly warned that this drug was capable of producing birth defects or even the death of the fetus, and stated that it should not be taken by women during pregnancy. Even so, a number of cases of congenital malformation have been reported in fetuses born to women using the drug. There is, of course, no positive way of knowing whether these were due to the tretinoin. Congenital malformations and spontaneous abortions were also occurring in women who were not taking or using tretinoin. Reports, in the popular press, of very large numbers of cases of malformations were almost certainly exaggerated. Interestingly, a study reported in the *Lancet* in May 1993 showed that the number of major fetal abnormalities occurring in pregnant women using tretinoin preparations on the skin was the same as the number in women not using the drug. Even so, if you are pregnant, better be safe than sorry.

Malignant Melanoma

In the last 40 years or so there has been a dramatic increase in the number of cases of the highly dangerous skin tumour malignant melanoma. There is now some evidence that antioxidant treatment with tretinoin can reduce this risk. Trials have suggested that the vitamin can normalize the early changes in the pigment cells (the *melanocytes*) that can progress to melanoma. They also suggest that tretinoin can retard the growth of melanomas and reduce their tendency to spread remotely. This research is still in an early stage.

If there is one lesson to be learned from all this, it is that prevention is better than cure. Sunbathing is a very bad habit. If you must do it, you should be quite sure that your skin is adequately protected by an effective sunscreen preparation.

Stroke

Stroke is the devastating consequence of a loss of the blood supply to a part of the brain so that damage occurs and the affected person is deprived, often permanently, of the full use of one or more of the brain functions — movement, sensation, speech, comprehension, vision and so on. Threatened strokes are called *transient ischaemic attacks* (TIAs). These are mini-strokes lasting for less than 24 hours and then, apparently, reversing. Any of the manifestations of a full stroke may occur and TIAs are clear indications that one is at risk.

The *Lancet* for 27 June 1992 carried a paper from the Department of Neurology at Brussels University, describing a study of 80 people who were showing definite signs of being at severe risk of developing a stroke. In this study, patients with TIAs lasting for more than three hours were matched against similar people who had never had TIAs, and the outcome assessed after 21 days. It was found that people with more than average vitamin A in their blood were significantly more likely to make a complete recovery than those with average amounts or less. Levels of vitamin E were also assessed but no significant difference was found between those with below or above average concentrations of this vitamin. The trial indicated that a high concentration of vitamin A in the blood produced a beneficial effect on the outcome. It also showed that those people whose symptoms and signs persisted for more than 24 hours, and whose blood levels of vitamin A were higher than average, ended up with less neurological damage than did those with low blood concentrations of the vitamin.

Destruction of nerve cells in stroke and pre-stroke conditions is known to be partly due to oxidative damage by free radicals. The body does what it can to protect against these free radicals, but its capacity to do so is limited. We know that vitamin E is highly effective as a free radical 'mop' in the presence of high concentrations of oxygen. Stroke and TIAs occur because blood is not getting through to carry oxygen to the nerve cells. This may be why vitamin E seems ineffective in this case. Vitamin A, on the other hand, is a powerful antioxidant in conditions of low oxygen concentrations, and this may account for its apparent value in these cases. It is, of course, possible that it also has valuable effects other than simply free radical trapping.

A lesson to be learned from this study would seem to be that each antioxidant has its optimum range of action, and that several different antioxidants are needed to ensure comprehensive cover. It would be foolish in the extreme, however, to suppose that taking antioxidant vitamins is an effective substitute for a healthy life-style that minimizes the risk factors for stroke — smoking, overweight, a high saturated fat diet, low vegetable and fruit intake, and lack of exercise.

Free Radicals and Parkinson's Disease

Parkinson's disease, or *paralysis agitans*, is a progressively disabling condition featuring shaking of the hands with 'pill-rolling' finger movements, rigidity of muscles, slowness of speech and movements, difficulty in getting started in walking, tottering steps, a mask-like face and tiny handwriting. It is due to the degeneration of certain cells in the central part of the brain known as the *substantia nigra* that produce a substance called dopamine, and it is treated with the drug levodopa and other substances that stimulate dopamine receptors in the brain. The cause of the changes in the brain cells is unknown, but in the late 1980s it became clear that various oxidative processes involving the formation of free radicals were involved.

A large trial was therefore started in 1987 to see whether

vitamin E in doses of 2,000 mg per day could delay the progress of the disease. Eight hundred patients with Parkinson's disease were involved in the trial, which was conducted simultaneously in a large number of different hospitals and research departments in America and Canada. The patients were divided into four groups, one of which received the vitamin E. The trial report was published in 1993 in the *New England Journal of Medicine*.

Unhappily, the trial showed no evidence of any beneficial effect of vitamin E on the progress of the disease. According to the researchers, this disappointing result might have been due to the fact that inadequate amounts of the vitamin were able to pass the 'blood–brain barrier' to reach the cells of the *substantia nigra*. It was also suggested that a negative result with vitamin E did not necessarily imply that other antioxidants might also be ineffective. It suggested that trials of these were still warranted. There were no significant adverse effects attributable to the dosage of the vitamin. One of the groups in the trial was treated with another drug, deprenyl (selegiline). This group did enjoy worthwhile benefit in terms of slowing of the disease.

Medical research can benefit from its failures as well as its successes. This major study teaches that theoretical ideas about free radicals are not always borne out in practice. The demonstration that free radicals are the cause of a particular kind of cell damage does not necessarily mean that any one particular antioxidant taken by mouth will prevent such damage. The antioxidant has to be appropriate and it has to get to the site of free radical damage.

Dupuytren's Contracture of the Hand

Just to show that free radicals have been implicated in seemingly unlikely conditions, and that research into such conditions can throw light on the whole subject, I thought I would include this one. Dupuytren's contracture is a thickening and shortening of the fibrous layer below the skin of the palm of the hand, the *palmar fascia*, that leads to a fixed bending of the fingers into the palm, usually starting with the ring finger. It is surprisingly common, affecting between 4 and 6 per cent of middle-aged men, rising to about 20 per cent of men over 65.

In November 1987 Dr G. A. C. Murrell and colleagues of the Nuffield Department of Orthopaedic Surgery, Oxford University, published a paper in the *British Medical Journal* reporting the results of the measurement of free radical markers in samples of damaged palmar fascia removed at operation on patients with Dupuytren's contracture. The free radical markers were hypoxanthine and xanthine, substances known to be implicated in the production of oxygen free radicals. Samples of normal fascia were obtained, to act as controls, from patients who did not have Dupuytren's contracture, but who were undergoing similar tissue removal operations for a different reason.

The samples taken from the Dupuytren's cases had six times the concentration of hypoxanthine as the control samples from people without Dupuytren's contracture. The researchers also confirmed the presence of the enzyme xanthine oxidase, which, acting on hypoxanthine, produces free radicals. All this strongly suggested that free radicals were the cause of the contracture. The scientists went further, however, and in laboratory experiments on tissue cultures of cells from the samples, showed that adding free radicals in appropriate concentration caused the cells to increase greatly in number. These cells are called *fibroblasts* and it is they that produce the additional scar tissue that causes the contracture. Free radicals in excess killed the cells.

The drug allopurinol is known to be valuable in the

management of Dupuytren's contracture. This drug acts by binding to the enzyme xanthine oxidase so that it cannot act on hypoxanthine to release free radicals.

Free Radicals and AIDS

It is interesting to note that people who are HIV positive and are showing signs of AIDS have a much higher incidence of Dupuytren's contracture than HIV-negative people. In a study of a series of examinations of 50 HIV-positive men, published in the *British Medical Journal* in 1990, 18 (36 per cent) had established Dupuytren's contracture and another 6 were thought to have early thickening of the palm.

One plausible reason for this extraordinarily high incidence of the condition in HIV-positive people may be that free radicals are produced in excessive amounts in such individuals. Increased amounts of the free radical marker malonaldehyde (see p.38) has indeed been found in people with HIV infection. This was reported in the *Scandinavian Journal of Infectious Diseases* in 1988.

Phagocytes and Free Radicals

Phagocytes (literally 'eating cells') are the scavengers of the body and do a wonderful job eating up and destroying undesirable substances and germs. They are mobile cells that are attracted to the site of infections or to foreign material by chemical stimuli. They get around by putting out long finger-like protrusions ('false feet' or *pseudopodia*) and flowing into them. This mobility also allows them to flow around anything they wish to destroy so that it is incorporated into their bodies. Inside the phagocytes are enzymes which, in the presence of bacteria and other organisms, produce the powerful oxygen free radical *superoxide*. This immediately generates the strong oxidant *hydrogen peroxide*. Hydrogen peroxide then acts on chloride in the phagocyte to form hypochlorous acid (the same stuff as Domestos), which soon copes with the germs.

Long-term inflammation means that successive waves of millions of phagocytes descend on the affected area of the body. Unfortunately, the free radicals do not stay in the phagocytes and large quantities are released into the surrounding tissues. Hydrogen peroxide and hypochlorous acid are profoundly damaging to body cells of all kinds and this is why inflammation is associated with tissue destruction. They also inflict damage on DNA and so can lead to cancer.

Red Wine and Free Radicals

Doctors have, for years, been embarrassed when asked why it is that the French, whose diet is high in saturated fats, nevertheless have a low incidence of the serious arterial disease atherosclerosis and a correspondingly low mortality from coronary heart disease. In medical circles, this is known as the 'French paradox'. Some medical men, especially those with a taste for wine, have maintained that this can somehow be attributed to a regular intake of red wine. The reasons they have given for this opinion have usually referred to the artery-widening (vasodilatation) effect of the alcohol content of the wine, and have not been found particularly plausible. A better suggestion has now been produced.

In the *British Medical Journal* of 20 February 1993 a paper appeared by scientists of the Lipid Research Group of the University of California. This paper refers to the previous research that showed how oxidation of the cholesterol-carrying low-density lipoproteins (LDLs) allows cholesterol to be incorporated into the plaques of atherosclerosis in the walls of arteries (see pp.18—20).

The paper then turns to a consideration of certain of the non-alcoholic constituents of the wine — several phenolic substances (*flavonoids*) which are known to have antioxidant properties. Phenolics were prepared from Californian red wine and tested for their antioxidant powers on human low-density lipoproteins in the laboratory. These tests showed that the phenolic substances were even more effective than vitamin E in preventing the oxidation of LDLs. Wine diluted one thousand-fold, containing tiny quantities of phenolics, inhibited oxidation of LDLs significantly more than vitamin E. According to the authors, 'These data provide a plausible explanation for the French paradox . . .'

Adult Respiratory Distress Syndrome and Free Radicals

The respiratory distress syndrome of adults is a serious and previously unpredictable complication of severe infection in which the lungs fill up with fluid and white cells and there is severe, often fatal, interference with the vital oxygenation of the blood. Recent research has shown that in this condition the balance of power between free radicals and natural body antioxidants changes in favour of the free radicals.

A report in the *Lancet* in March 1993 shows that measurements of certain of the body's natural antioxidants makes it possible to identify which people are most likely to develop this dangerous syndrome so that preventive treatment can be given. This study showed that 9 to 12 hours before the syndrome developed, the people concerned showed a definite rise in the amounts of superoxide dismutase and catalase (see p.12) present in their bodies. This is a clear indication of increased free radical activity, giving warning of impending trouble. Since free radicals are now implicated in so many different conditions it seems likely that anticipatory investigations of this kind may become more important in the future.

The Expansion of Medical Interest in Free Radicals

This paper is just another example of the reports of free radical research now appearing with increasing regularity in the professional medical press. Other conditions in which free radicals have been implicated or suspected of being important include pressure sores, red blood cell damage, paraquat poisoning, carbon tetrachloride poisoning, ozone damage, skeletal muscle damage, liver cell damage, spinal cord injury, diabetes and possibly even cancer caused by electromagnetic fields from power lines. They have also been found to be active in alcohol toxicity and in bringing about the destructive action of anticancer drugs.

Papers on free radicals have appeared in numerous medical and other journals from all over the world. Here are a few, in addition to those already mentioned, that have published on the subject: *Annals of the Royal College of Surgeons of England, Journal of the American College of Cardiology, Nature, Journal of Biological Chemistry, Cancer Research, American Journal of Clinical Nutrition, Journal of Pharmacology, Biochemical Medicine, American Journal of Epidemiology, Toxicology and Applied Pharmacology, Annals of Clinical Biochemistry, Acta Physiologica Scandinavica, Gastroenterology, International Journal of Epidemiology, Journal of*

Inorganic Biochemistry and the journal *Free Radical Biology and Medicine.*

With this much serious medical and scientific interest in the subject, can you afford to ignore it?

9

What are Antioxidants?

An antioxidant is any substance that retards or prevents deterioration, damage or destruction by oxidation. As we have seen in Chapter 1, free radicals act by oxidation. Oxidation is always damaging to whatever is oxidized, although often it is very useful — indeed, it is the source of all our energy, and our bodies could not work without it. But in other cases, as when free radicals bring about cell damage in disease processes, it is far from useful and we naturally want to try to do something to stop it. This is where *antioxidants* come in. In a medical context, they are comparatively new, but in other branches of science they have been around for a long time.

Antioxidants

For many years, chemists have known that free radical oxidation action can be controlled or even prevented by a range of antioxidant substances. It is, for instance, vital that lubricating oils should remain stable and liquid and should not dry up like paints. For this reason, such oils usually have small quantities of antioxidants, such as phenol or amine derivatives, added to them. Although plastics are often formed by free radical action, they can also be broken down by the same process. So they, too, require protection by antioxidants like phenols or naphthols. Low-density polythene is also often protected by carbon black which absorbs the ultraviolet light which causes free radical production (see p.54).

Food in storage also deteriorates by oxidation. When, for instance, fat goes rancid it does so by a free radical oxidation reaction. Oxidized fats are new compounds that taste and smell horrible and anything that can prevent this happening is of great economic importance. So chemists have for some time been actively looking for antioxidants for this purpose. To date, the most popular antioxidant food additives have been BHA (butylated hydroxyanisole), BHT (butylated hydroxytoluene), propyl gallate and tocopherol (vitamin E). These antioxidants act by donating hydrogen atoms to the hydroxyl radical so that water is formed. The equation is simple: $H + OH = H_2O$. In other words, two dangerously active radicals combine to form a harmless molecule: water.

Ironically, the irradiation of food — which is an excellent way of killing bacteria that can cause spoilage and may be dangerous — can, in itself, cause free radical production that can lead to unacceptable chemical changes in the food. So it may sometimes be necessary to counteract the undesirable effects of irradiation of food by using antioxidants.

Natural Body Antioxidants

Fortunately, the body has its own antioxidants for damage limitation. One of the most effective of these is the substance tocopherol (vitamin E). This vitamin dissolves in fat and that is especially important because by far the most significant free radical damage in the body is damage to the membranes of cells and to low-density lipoproteins, and these are made of fat molecules. Vitamin C is also a powerful antioxidant, but is soluble in water, not in fat. This means that it gets distributed to all parts of the body. The two vitamins are both highly efficient at mopping up free radicals, and sometimes even co-operate in so doing.

Other natural body antioxidants include compounds such as *cysteine*, *glutathione* and *D-penicillamine*, and blood constituents such as the iron-containing molecule *transferrin* and the protein *ceruloplasmin*. These act either by preventing free radicals from being produced or by mopping them up.

As mentioned in Chapter 1, the body also contains a number of important antioxidant *enzymes*. An enzyme is a highly active protein that accelerates a chemical reaction. Most of what goes on in the body is promoted by thousands of different enzymes. The most interesting antioxidant enzyme is *superoxide dismutase*. This excited enormous interest when it was discovered, as it has no other function than to change the dangerous superoxide free radical to the safer hydrogen peroxide. This made the scientists think and really got the doctors interested in free radicals. Hydrogen peroxide (H_2O_2), although not a free radical, is not particularly pleasant stuff to have around. The extra oxygen atom is readily available to cause oxidation, making it an active compound useful for producing blonde hair. So the body has two other enzymes, *catalase* and *glutathione peroxidase* that break down hydrogen peroxide to water and oxygen.

Vitamins

The greatest popular interest, however, is currently focused on the vitamins. Most current medical textbooks still treat vitamins, including vitamin C and vitamin E, in the conventional manner, by giving small recommended daily allowances (RDAs). This is appropriate for the large B group of vitamins (B1, B2, B6 and B12, niacin, pantothenic acid, folic acid and lipoic acid) and for vitamins D and K. All these, plus vitamin C, are substances necessary in very small quantities for the maintenance of health. If these small quantities are not available, various deficiency diseases occur. Vitamin C deficiency causes scurvy, a bleeding disorder; vitamin A deficiency causes serious eye and other problems; vitamin D deficiency causes bone softening, rickets or osteomalacia; and so on.

Danger of Overdosage

Because many vitamins act in association with enzymes and only tiny quantities are required, it has become conventional to teach that people who take more than the small daily requirement — which is nearly always present in a reasonably balanced diet — are wasting their money. In addition, there have been regular, and well-justified, medical warnings about the dangers of vitamin overdosage, specifically of vitamins A and D. Excessive intake of these vitamins can certainly cause trouble. Too much vitamin D causes calcium to be deposited in the kidneys, arteries and other tissues — a serious matter that can lead to all sorts of problems, including kidney failure. The dangers of vitamin A overdosage are described below, as are those of vitamin E.

Although few textbooks have yet got around to the role of certain vitamins as biological antioxidants, there is plenty about this in current medical and general scientific literature. Textbooks take a long time to write, edit and publish and they invariably lag behind current advances, especially in new and rapidly developing fields of research. This is why medical and scientific journals are so important. In the free radical literature most of the emphasis has been on vitamins E and C, so it will be worth looking more closely at these interesting substances.

Vitamin E (Tocopherol)

Until recently, pharmacology textbooks have dismissed the fat-soluble vitamin E as unimportant; some have even said that it is of no medical relevance in humans.

Tocopherol was first discovered in 1922 when it was found that female rats required an unknown substance in their diets to sustain normal pregnancies. Without it, they could ovulate and conceive satisfactorily, but within about 10 days the fetus invariably died and was absorbed. Male rats deficient in this substances were also found to have abnormalities in their testes. For these reasons, vitamin E enjoyed a brief reputation as the 'antisterility vitamin' and was, illogically, recommended as a treatment for infertility, although there was no reason to suppose that the people concerned were deficient in the vitamin. It has also been used to try to treat various menstrual disorders, inflammation of the vagina and menopausal symptoms, but there is no reason to suppose that it is specifically useful in these conditions.

Vitamin E was first isolated in 1936 from wheat germ oil. It was found to be any one of a range of eight very complicated but similar molecules known as tocopherols. It is almost insoluble in water but dissolves in oils, fats, alcohol, acetone, ether and other fat solvents. Unlike vitamin C it is stable to heat and alkalis in the absence of oxygen and is unaffected by acids at temperatures up to 100° C. If exposed to atmospheric oxygen it is slowly oxidized. This occurs more rapidly in the presence of iron or silver salts. It gradually darkens on exposure to light. Among the richest natural sources are seed germ oils, alfalfa and lettuce. It is widely distributed in plant materials. The international unit is equal to 1 mg of alpha-tocopherol acetate. For practical purposes of dosage, consider 1 international unit to be equivalent to 1 mg.

All the tocopherols are antioxidants and this appears to be the basis for all the biological effects of the vitamin. It is now becoming increasingly clear that vitamin E operates as a natural antioxidant helping to protect important cell structures, especially the cell membranes, from the damaging effects of free radicals. Interestingly, it has been found, for instance, that the vitamin can protect against the effects of overdosage of vitamin A described below. It is involved in many body processes.

In carrying out its function as an antioxidant in the body, vitamin E is, itself, converted to a radical. It is, however, soon regenerated to the active vitamin by a biochemical process that probably involves both vitamin C and glutathione.

Deficiency of vitamin E is very rare because it occurs widely in food, especially in vegetable oils, but when it does occur the effects can be devastating. The need for vitamin E increases if the diet is high in polyunsaturated fats. Deficiency sometimes occurs in premature babies, especially if malnourished, and in people with disorders that interfere with fat absorption. People who are severely deficient in vitamin E for these reasons may suffer, to varying degrees, degenerative changes in the brain and nervous system, impairment of vision, double vision, walking disturbances, anaemia, an increased rate of destruction of red blood cells, fluid retention (oedema) and skin disorders. Some reports have shown that large doses of vitamin E can prevent the progression of the neurological abnormalities or even lead to improvement.

Human vitamin E deficiency occurs only after many months on a severely deficient diet. A daily intake of 10 to

30 mg of the vitamin is said to be sufficient to keep the blood levels within normal limits and this will always be provided by a normal diet. Diets that contain other antioxidants decrease the requirement. Human milk contains plenty to meet the baby's needs.

Dangers of overdosage

Vitamin E is generally regarded as being a fairly innocuous substance and few if any warnings are heard of the dangers of overdosage. For adults, this is probably reasonable, but there are undoubtedly limits to the amounts that can be safely taken. Dangers have arisen from overdosage of vitamin E in premature babies from probable interference with the action of cells of the immune system against infection (see p.56). Since free radical oxidant action is a necessary part of the body's functioning, both for the destruction of bacteria and for other important purposes, it is only reasonable to suppose that undue interference with it, by excessive dosage of an antioxidant like vitamin E, is likely to be harmful. To do so may be, for instance, to increase the risk of infection.

There is no substance of major medical benefit that does not also carry the risk of undesirable side effects. This is a fact of medical life that should never be forgotten. Like many other substances, vitamin E is necessary for life and health. But, like many other substances, the amount in the body must, for safety, be kept within fairly strict limits.

Vitamin C (Ascorbic Acid)

Vitamin C is a simpler compound than vitamin E and is water-soluble. It was the first vitamin to be discovered, and the disease caused by its deficiency — scurvy — has been known for centuries. Sailors on long sea voyages, who subsisted on salt pork and biscuits, with no fresh fruit or vegetables, used commonly to die of scurvy. But in 1747, the British naval doctor James Lind (1716—84) proved by careful experiments, with controls, that a teaspoonful of lemon juice, taken from time to time, would prevent the disease. Unfortunately, it was 50 years before Their Lordships of the Admiralty — who were not readily impressed by science — could be persuaded to issue appropriate orders to their ships' captains, and in the meantime many more sailors died.

The vitamin was isolated in 1928 and chemically identified in 1932. It is readily destroyed by exposure to air and by cooking, especially in the presence of copper and alkalis. The main structural material of the body is a protein called collagen. This forms the main basis of the bones and of most other tissues. Vitamin C is necessary for the proper synthesis of collagen, and deficiency leads to the failure of wounds to heal, to weakness of small blood vessels with bleeding from the gums and into the joints and skin, to anaemia and looseness of the teeth. Scurvy still occurs in people who live on tea and buns and the first signs — usually swollen and bleeding gums and loose teeth, but in some cases spontaneous bruising on the lower thighs — appear three or four months after the last intake of the vitamin. In babies and small children scurvy also causes bleeding under the bone membranes, causing very tender swellings so that infants resent being touched.

To prevent scurvy, humans need amounts of vitamin C varying from about 60 mg a day to as much as 250 mg a day. Blood levels of the vitamin are reduced by smoking and by the contraceptive pill. People need more while suffering from infectious diseases, injuries, burns, rheumatic disorders and after surgical operations. A normal, well-balanced diet will usually supply enough vitamin C to prevent scurvy. The vitamin is plentiful in fruit juices, green peppers, cabbages, greens, potatoes, citrus fruits, tomatoes and strawberries. Orange and lemon juices contain about 0.5 mg in each cc (ml). When large doses are taken, there is a correspondingly large loss of the vitamin in the urine.

Vitamin C is a powerful antioxidant and for this reason is commonly used to preserve the natural flavour and colour of processed fruit, vegetables and dairy products.

The Value of Vitamin C in Medicine

No one disputes that vitamin C is of great value in the treatment of scurvy. As soon as the vitamin is given in adequate dosage, improvement occurs and, within a few weeks, all the symptoms and signs have gone. The real dispute has been whether the vitamin has any value in people who are *not* suffering from scurvy. Until recently, the orthodox medical view has been that the vitamin does no good to such people. Oddly enough, in spite of this view, there have been, over the years, repeated enthusiasms for trials of the vitamin in all sorts of conditions. Even before the current interest in free radicals and in the use of antioxidants, vitamin C had many respectable supporters. One reason for the medical scepticism is clear: most of the trials of vitamin C in the management of conditions like the common cold failed because the doses given were very little more than the minimum daily requirement to prevent scurvy. It is becoming clear that, used as an antioxidant, much larger doses than the minimum daily requirement are needed.

How Much is Safe?

On this question, Linus Pauling made an interesting point while considering vitamin C in an evolutionary context.

Assuming that early peoples must have eaten whatever they could get their hands on, he decided to work out how much vitamin C they would have taken in if, as must often have happened, the total daily calorie requirement (2,500 calories) was met from a single foodstuff. The results were surprising. If they had eaten enough peas and beans to get 2,500 calories, they would have taken in 1,000 mg of vitamin C. Vegetables with a low vitamin C content would have provided 1,200 mg; vegetables and fruits with an intermediate content would have provided 3,400 mg; high C foods like cabbage, cauliflower, chives and mustard greens would have provided 6,000 mg per day; and very high C foods like black currants, kale, parsley, peppers and broccoli would have provided no less than 12,000 mg per day.

Since humans evolved in an environment providing quantities of vitamin C of this order, Pauling inferred that the ideal daily intake for most adults should be somewhere in the range of 2,300 to 9,000 mg. The very large vitamin C intake throughout a large part of the evolutionary period implied that big doses of this vitamin should be regarded as 'natural'.

Possible Dangers

Vitamin C has an excellent safety record and has been taken in 1,000 mg plus doses by millions of people with no apparent disadvantage. To balance this, there has been a handful of reports of ill effects thought to be due to very large doses of the vitamin.

One of these was published in the *British Medical Journal* in March 1993. This paper reports the case of a 32-year-old HIV-positive man who developed generalized lymph node enlargement. He was advised by his doctors to start AZT treatment but refused and sought the advice of a medically qualified nutritionist. Investigation showed that he had a lower than normal blood level of the antioxidant glutathione and he was prescribed, among other things, glutathione supplements and a course of vitamin C to be given in a dosage of 40,000 mg, by intravenous injection, three times a week, plus 20,000 to 40,000 mg every day, by mouth. This huge dosage was continued for a month with no obvious change in his condition. The intravenous dose was then doubled to 80,000 mg. The next day he became breathless and feverish and his urine turned to a black colour, indicating that many red blood cells had broken down, releasing haemoglobin which was passing out in the urine, much in the manner of malarial 'blackwater fever'.

Investigation showed that this man had sickle cell trait and a comparatively rare genetic blood disorder known as glucose-6-phosphate dehydrogenase deficiency. This enzyme deficiency disorder makes red blood cells much more fragile than normal because of a shortage of the antioxidant glutathione which protects the red cells against free radical damage. Many drugs in common use can cause the red cells to break down in this condition. The patient was given lots of fluid to drink so as to flush through his kidneys and on the third day the urine was clear. He made a complete recovery from the red blood cell breakdown.

Vitamin C dosages of this order are exceptional and there are few remedies that can, with perfect safety, be taken in quantities of 20 or 30 times the customary dosage. The report does, however, indicate that there are some people who ought to be particularly cautious about taking any drug, even one as apparently safe as vitamin C.

Beta-Carotene

The antioxidant plant pigment beta-carotene is also known as provitamin A because it is converted into vitamin A (retinol and other forms) in the liver. It is found in whole milk, butter, cheese, egg yolk, liver, yellow and green vegetables and fish, especially in the liver. The same foods also contain a number of different carotene-like substances (carotenoids) that cannot be converted to vitamin A and so are wasted.

Retinol and its related substances have many important functions in the body. They are necessary for the growth and health of the surface and lining tissues and the bones; for the health of the immune system and for protection against cancer; for normal vision and for the health of the corneas; for protection against various skin diseases; and for protection of the skin against sunlight radiation and ageing changes. People deficient in retinoids suffer night blindness and dryness of the eyes (xerophthalmia). Babies may suffer devastating melting of the corneas of the eyes with permanent blindness. Severe deficiency is a common cause of death in small children after severe damage has been sustained by most systems of the body.

A normal, well-balanced diet will provide quite enough retinol to prevent any such effects. If taken as a dietary supplement, 1 mg per day is equivalent to the recommended daily allowance and this dose will probably double the amount needed to prevent deficiency.

Dangers of Overdosage

Very large doses of vitamin A cause chronic poisoning with skin dryness, itching and peeling; drowsiness, irritability and an irresistible desire to sleep; headache; loss of appetite; enlargement of the liver and spleen; and painful and tender swellings over the bones. The vitamin accumulates in the body and the effects take weeks to wear off. Eskimos and their husky dogs never eat polar bear liver (which contains huge quantities of vitamin A) because they know of these effects. A single gram of polar bear liver contains up to 12 mg of retinol — 12 times the minimum daily requirement. Vitamin A is also dangerous to the fetus if taken by the mother in doses of 7 to 12 mg a day during the first three months of pregnancy. This can cause congenital abnormalities.

Once again, here is a warning about the fallacy of believing that if something is good for you, a lot of it will be even better. This is often true, but you shouldn't count on it. In some cases, a lot is very much worse.

10

The Argument and the Challenge

You now have what I hope is a fair summary of the facts on free radicals and antioxidants. This is a very large subject and when writing a book of this kind it is very difficult to avoid bias. Nothing is easier than to deliberately select those reports and arguments that support a particular point of view and to ignore or play down those that do not. To do this is neither honest nor safe.

At the same time, it is impossible to research and study a subject as potentially important as this without forming opinions and taking up a position. You will have gathered that I have long been convinced of the importance of free radicals and of the value of antioxidant vitamin treatment. I am reasonably sure, however, that I have not made any claims that are not well supported by scientific evidence. One must, of course, take on trust the statements made in the various reports and made verbally by scientific enthusiasts. This is not so hazardous as you might think. Published scientific work is closely and critically scrutinized by many other scientists, especially those working in the same field, and the one thing they are looking for are claims or assertions that they think may not be backed up by convincing evidence. All really important findings are independently checked by repeated research, carried out by other people, and many papers are published to refute or confirm such work.

There is one form of bias that I can, happily, disclaim at once. You will be aware that major commercial interests are involved in a subject of this kind. If everyone starts taking daily doses of antioxidant vitamins, the people who make them are going to enjoy enormously increased profits. An already flourishing industry is going to expand many times. So let me declare at once that I am an independent free-lance writer, with no connection of any kind with any firm of pharmaceutical manufacturers. I am not implying by this that drug manufacturers go in for dishonest claims or try to promote books that make such claims; the pharmaceutical firms' publications are exposed to the same critical surveillance as any other serious scientific reports, and they greatly value their ethical status.

Be Sceptical

Having declared my interest, I am now going to summarize the arguments and challenge you to make up your own minds on the matter. I hope you will read what follows with scepticism. In particular, you should be wary of believing that just because something follows something else the second must necessarily be a consequence of the first. Let me give you an example of what I mean.

I used regularly to have colds, often every two or three weeks. Years ago, I started to take 1,000 mg of vitamin C every day and, whenever a cold seemed to be threatening, I increased the dosage to 2,000 or 3,000 mg daily. Since then I have had hardly any established colds and almost always find that I can abort a cold with the extra dosage. *This is not proof.* On this basis alone, I am not entitled to believe that it is the vitamin C that is preventing the colds. Other things may have happened, coincidentally with my starting to take the vitamin, that increased my resistance to colds. I might have changed my life-style in such a way as to come in contact with fewer people bearing cold germs. It is even possible that my expectation of benefit from vitamin C brings it about by some obscure psychological effect on my immune system.

But if, at the same time, I have evidence that the viruses that cause colds do so by producing free radicals (I don't actually know this, although I suspect that it is true), and that vitamin C can mop up free radicals, then I am entitled to have more confidence in the idea that vitamin C prevents colds. Since I have no evidence that viruses produce free radicals, I must continue to consider the matter 'not proven'.

The Romans recognized the logical fallacy of believing that because one event follows another the former must have been the cause of the latter. They called it the *post hoc ergo propter hoc* fallacy ('after this, therefore because of this'). This is one of the commonest forms of logical error, and we are all prone to it.

With this warning in mind, here is a brief summary of the facts presented so far.

The Argument

Cells are the tiny, microscopic units of which the body is made. They are living, highly active units, busily engaged in carrying out thousands of chemical reactions concerned with energy production, protein synthesis, growth and repair, material storage, information transmission, hormone production, detoxification of poisons and drugs, and so on. Similar cells join together to form simple tissues, these form more complex tissues, tissues form organs, and organs form systems.

Disease is any impairment of the structure or the function

of cells. So it can affect single cells, tissues, organs, whole systems or the whole body. Until comparatively recently, the actual way in which the molecules of body cells are injured in disease was unknown. We knew a great deal about the changes that occur in cells in the course of disease but little about the way in which this was brought about. We also knew how important the outer layer of the cell — the cell membrane — was, and how often disease processes resulted in damage to this membrane. The cell membrane is made mainly of cholesterol, a form of fat. We also knew that disease processes damage other parts of the cell, including the tiny cell organs (organelles) such as the mitochondria that produce energy, and the DNA at the centre of the cell (the nucleus).

We now know that a very important way in which cell membranes and other parts of the cell can be damaged is by the chemical reactions that occur between the molecules of the cell and a class of short-lived but highly active chemical groups known as oxygen free radicals (see pp.6–7, 11). This chemical reaction is known as oxidation — a kind of burning — and it is always damaging to the substances oxidized (see pp.7–8). Free radicals also convert normal body molecules into free radicals and thus often start chain reactions which multiply the damage (see p.8).

A later discovery was that the body has its own, built-in systems for combating free radicals. These are normal body constituents, known as antioxidants (see p.81), and their function is to get rid of excess free radicals. They do this by altering them slightly so that they cease to be chemically active and become harmless. More than half a dozen of these natural antioxidants are known (see p.82). One of them is vitamin E, usually called alpha-tocopherol (see pp.85–7). It is very rare for anyone to be severely deficient in vitamin E, but when this happens, almost every part of the body suffers serious damage. The killing and scavenging cells of our immune system (phagocytes) use free radicals to destroy the germs they have absorbed. At least in very small babies, too much vitamin E can interfere with this action and allow infection to get the upper hand (see p.87). So we know that in some cases it is possible to have too much vitamin E.

Vitamin E does not dissolve in water but does dissolve in fat. Cell membranes and low-density lipoproteins (see pp.18—19) are largely made of the fatty material cholesterol. Vitamin E is probably the only antioxidant that can fix itself to cell membranes and to LDLs. So it seems probable that this is the main protective substance against cell membrane and LDL oxidation damage.

The body also reacts badly to a deficiency of vitamin C (see pp.87—8) but the effects of this are much less widespread than those of a deficiency of vitamin E. Vitamin C, however, is a powerful antioxidant and is soluble in water, so it makes its way to every part of the body, which is over 90 per cent water. All the cells of the body contain water and all are bathed in water. The amount of vitamin C in the body varies considerably with the diet and doses up to about 10,000 mg a day are probably harmless (see pp.89—90).

Many hundreds of medical and scientific papers have now been published showing that various disease conditions are associated with free radicals. Hundreds have also been published showing that if the body is low in antioxidants, especially vitamin E, vitamin C and beta-carotene (see pp.91—3), the affected person is more likely to suffer from various diseases. So far, the strongest evidence is in connection with the serious artery disease atherosclerosis (see p.14), which causes heart attacks, strokes and gangrene, and is the largest single cause of death in the Western world. Free radicals have actually been detected following heart attacks (see p.25). There is also convincing evidence that low antioxidant levels promote the eye disease cataract.

Good evidence also exists that free radicals are strongly implicated in the cellular changes occurring in ageing, in the damage caused by smoking and in the destructive effects of sunlight on the skin. We know that free radicals can damage DNA and there are grounds, less secure than for other conditions, for the belief that they are implicated in the development of at least some cancers. Low antioxidant levels in men are associated with increased birth defects in their children.

Cigarette smoking causes a substantial drop in the levels of antioxidants in the bodies of smokers (see p.66). This is believed to be because cigarette smoke contains so many free radicals and promotes so many additional free radicals in the body that much of the antioxidant potential is used up coping with these. As a result, cigarette smokers are more heavily under attack from free radicals than non-smokers. There is a wealth of evidence for the view that the wide spectrum of increased disease and premature mortality suffered by smokers is largely due to the action of free radicals.

The Challenge

The obvious next stage is to carry out trials to see whether heart disease, stroke, cancer, cataract and so on can actually be prevented by taking antioxidant vitamins. This is not as straightforward as it sounds, as it is impossible to tell for certain whether someone is going to be spared such diseases until they are actually dead. Such trials, therefore, must inevitably take many years. Many major trials have, however, already started and there is nothing for it but to wait patiently. This is where the challenge comes in. Unless you are very young, there is not much point is waiting ten years or so for proof that you should have been doing something really important for years. You really have to make up your mind *now*.

If the scientific researchers — many from the world's most prestigious research institutions and universities — are wrong, and this free radical business is all nonsense, then you do have quite a lot to lose. Financially, the cost of 1,000—2,000 mg of vitamin C and 200—400 mg of vitamin E a day is perhaps £10 every month — maybe less if you shop around. Vitamin C is very cheap, but unless done up in coated tablets or in a flavoured, fizzy formulation, is horribly sour and you may soon get discouraged. The fancy preparations are, unfortunately, much more expensive than the basic acid.

Medically, the likelihood of any harmful side effects of such dosage is quite slight, as millions of people have already proved, but it is possible that the very occasional sensitive person might show what is called an *idiosyncratic reaction* of some kind. Such things do happen. If you do notice any such harmful effect, stop the tablets and capsules. You will also have to watch your intake of vitamin A — not by taking lots of pills, which could be dangerous, but by ensuring that your diet is adequately rich in A (see p.92).

But suppose it is true that free radicals are, at this very moment, attacking and oxidizing your low-density lipoproteins so that they are damaging the walls of your arteries, clogging them up with atheromatous plaques and cutting down the vital blood supply to your heart, brain, other organs and limbs. It is true that whenever you are exposed to sunlight, the collagen in your skin is being attacked and degraded by radiation-induced free radicals so that it can no longer maintain youthful smoothness and elasticity or provide the support that prevents wrinkling and broken veins. It is true that, as you read, the protein in the internal lenses of your eyes is being oxidized and changed so that cataracts may form. Perhaps worst of all, it is true that the DNA in many of the cells of your body is being attacked and damaged by free radicals so that the race is on between the rate of damage and the processes of repair. If the free radicals win, the result may simply be the death of some cells, which is of no great consequence. But it may also be a DNA mutation that could proceed to a cancerous change in a cell or, in the case of the sperm-producing cells, a genetic mutation that could be passed on to the children.

So it is up to you.

One last and very important point. If you are convinced that this kind of self-treatment actually does work, you might be tempted to use it as a substitute for healthy living, and especially as a justification for continuing to smoke. You could hardly make a more serious mistake. Antioxidant treatment may well turn out to be of major health importance, but it can never be a substitute for a healthy life-style.

Questions and Answers about Free Radicals and Antioxidants

Are people who don't eat leafy green and yellow vegetables more liable to suffer certain diseases, such as cancer, than people who do?
The evidence of a number of surveys certainly suggests so.

Is this because of the protective effect of antioxidant vitamins?
That is the general presumption.

Why do textbooks of nutrition recommend doses of vitamins C and E that are so much smaller than those you are recommending?
The textbooks are concerned simply with avoiding the vitamin-deficiency diseases. Few have yet got around to recognizing the value of antioxidant vitamins as general health measures. This is a basically different use of these vitamins.

Would it be a good thing to take much larger doses of vitamin D and the B vitamins as well?
On no account should you take large doses of vitamin D — or of vitamin A for that matter. Both would be dangerous (see p.84). The B vitamins are not antioxidants. They are co-enzymes, needed to allow various body enzyme systems to work and are needed in very small quantities. You will get no advantage from taking larger doses than the recommended minimum daily allowances and you will get these from a decent balanced diet.

Which vitamins are fat-soluble?
Vitamins A, D, E and K are fat-soluble; C is water-soluble.

Does the solubility matter?
Yes. Fat-soluble antioxidants stay in cell membranes, which are made of two layers of fat molecules, and in low-density lipoproteins. Water-soluble vitamins may be present in the water in the cell or in the water surrounding the cell, but not in the membrane. Remember that antioxidants must get very close to the point of free radical production if they are to work.

What happens when free radicals attack a cell membrane?
Hydroxyl free radicals have a voracious appetite for electrons and immediately hunt out unsaturated (double) bonds in the fatty acids of the membrane fats. When one of these bonds is broken, the molecule is split and the parts will have unpaired electrons (see p.2). That means that they are now, themselves, free radicals. These, in turn, attack other fatty acid bonds, so a chain reaction can zip through the cell membrane causing terrible damage and even killing the cell.

Which free radicals does vitamin E deal with – the original cause of the chain reaction or those in the membrane?
Vitamin E copes with both, but is especially important in blocking cell membrane chain reactions. It is a brilliant scavenger of split fat molecule free radicals, and does a great job in stopping chain reactions and saving cells.

How does vitamin E work?
Vitamin E, being fat-soluble, settles in cell membranes and in low-density lipoproteins (see pp.18—19). Its molecule carries a hydroxyl group (see p.6) from which the hydrogen atom is easily removed. This contributes the single electron

needed to fill the outer orbital of any nearby free radical and render it harmless. This, of course, turns the vitamin E molecule into a free radical, but apparently it can move to the surface of the cell membrane or LDL globule where it reacts with vitamin C and is restored to normal.

Does this mean that if we are taking vitamin E, we should also take vitamin C?
Yes. But I believe we should be taking C, anyhow, for all sorts of other reasons.

Vitamin E doses are given in IU not mg. What are IU?
International units. Vitamin E, in practice, is not a pure substance but a mixture of tocopherols, of which there are eight or so. You will not go far wrong if you count international units as mg (milligrams). A milligram of alpha-tocopherol acetate — the commonest form — is equal to an international unit.

How much vitamin C should we take?
No one knows for sure. However, although the present official recommended minimum daily allowance is probably enough to stop you from getting scurvy, it isn't going to be much good for anything else. In certain circumstances it might not even prevent scurvy. The trouble is that the body's antioxidant needs are constantly changing. If your cells are under especial attack because of an infection or because you are on certain drugs or have inhaled a lot of car exhaust fumes or because you are a smoker, or even because you have accidentally taken some poisonous substance, then you will need a lot more than the basic amount — whatever that is. The big trials currently under way should show what sort of dosage can cover most eventualities. I suspect that 1,000 mg a day should be considered a minimum and that you should take 2,000 mg or 3,000 mg if you think you are at risk.

What do you mean, 'at risk'?
If you get a slight sore throat or any other indication of a cold, increase the daily dose. Similarly, if you feel unwell and suspect that you are 'sickening' for something. The time may come when we will up the intake for any early sign of indisposition or minor injury of any kind. Don't imagine, however, that an extra dose of vitamin C is any substitute for proper medical attention when this is obviously needed. Solid vitamin C tablets are also probably not a very good idea if you suffer from peptic ulcers or severe dyspepsia. In such cases, use a soluble preparation.

I understand the body stores vitamin C. Is this true?
Yes. Most people who are not taking supplementary vitamin C have a store of about 1,500 mg or more. If you take an additional daily dose, the store will reach about 2,500 mg and you will start to pass more vitamin C in the urine. To maintain a store of 2,500 mg requires an intake of more than this amount every day. It is possible that the blood and tissue levels associated with a 2,500 mg store will cope with most free radical problems, but this is not certain. The more that is taken, the higher the levels of the vitamin in the blood and the tissue fluids. We excrete more vitamin C if the intake is such as to raise the body's vitamin C content above the 2,500 mg level, but this does not imply that one cannot raise the amount above this level.

Is it true that some animals make their own vitamin C?
Yes. In fact, only humans, the apes and other primates, guinea pigs and some bats are unable to synthesize vitamin C. Animals make it from glucose, but we lack the liver enzyme to carry out the last stage in the process. This suggests that earlier in evolution we were able to make the vitamin but that a mutation occurred in the common

ancestor of the primates, maybe around 25,000,000 years ago, so that the gene for this enzyme was deleted.

What are carotenoids?
These are the substances found in plants, fish liver, other liver, dairy products, etc. that are converted by the human liver into vitamin A. Beta-carotene is the most active carotenoid found in plants. There is growing evidence that, quite apart from their role as provitamin A, carotenoids can prevent, or help to prevent, various diseases.

Can they prevent cancer?
It is not certain. There is plenty of statistical evidence that if you take a large group of people all with high levels of beta-carotene in their blood and compare them with an equal group with low levels of beta-carotene, the first group will have fewer cases of cancer than the second, especially lung cancer. This has been reported in the *British Journal of Cancer* and in the medical journal *Cancer*. This doesn't, however, prove that beta-carotene prevents cancer. It does seem likely that it decreases your chances of getting some kinds of cancer.

Is taking beta-carotene the same as taking vitamin A?
Not quite. Although the two are closely related chemically, beta-carotene has been shown to have value against free radicals in certain conditions in which vitamin A seems ineffective. Beta-carotene is, however, the main human source of vitamin A and is soon converted by the liver into vitamin A, but this takes different forms with different functions. One form (retinal) is necessary for vision, others (retinol, retinoic acid, etc.) are necessary for healthy surface tissues (epithelia), and so on.

Appendix 1

How does beta-carotene reduce the risk of some types of cancer? Is this an antioxidant effect?

Very likely. Beta-carotene is a powerful antioxidant that mops up free radicals produced by radiation or by various cancer-producing substances (carcinogens). These free radicals can cause DNA mutations that can lead to cancer. Moreover, a shortage of beta-carotene has, for some time, been known to lead to particular changes in surface cells (epithelia) characteristic of early cancer. The administration of beta-carotene reverses these early changes.

There seems to be some evidence that fields from electric power lines and transformers can cause cancer. Could a free radical with its unpaired electron be affected by such fields?

Yes. Very weak fields of the strength caused by power lines, etc., could move free radicals and, at least in theory, might interfere with pairs of radicals with opposite electron spin hooking up with each other to form a safe, non-active, pair. If this happened on a large scale there would be far more free radicals about than normal and this could lead to cancer.

It's all very theoretical and I don't think there has been any proof that this actually happens. Don't forget that all of us have been exposed to the earth's magnetic field from the time of conception. Maybe the interaction of the fixed field of the earth and the alternating field from power lines could have undesirable effects. The chemist Keith McLauchlan of Oxford University published a paper on this in January 1992 in *Physics World*.

What happens when molecules are oxidized?

First, a couple of oxygen atoms, linked together to form an oxygen molecule, approach the target molecule. Then an electron is transferred from the target molecule onto the oxygen molecule. This turns the oxygen molecule into a superoxide free radical, avid to link onto something. And, of course, the thing it latches onto is the target molecule, changing it to a quite different compound — an oxide.

In what way different?
As different as rust is from iron or quicklime is from chalk, or laughing gas is from nitrogen. Oxides have quite different properties from the parent substance before it was oxidized.

But oxidation is essential to life. Does this mean that superoxide free radicals are essential too?
Yes. But the enzyme that makes them safe — superoxide dismutase (see pp.12, 83) — is also essential to life. This has been shown by experiments in which bacteria were genetically engineered so that the gene for superoxide dismutase was removed. They couldn't take it and they all died.

Has there ever been a case reported of a deficiency of superoxide dismutase in humans?
`Not that I know of. This would almost certainly be a lethal mutation causing death at a very early stage after conception.

How is it possible to detect free radicals?
Free radicals have a single unpaired electron in the outer orbital. The paired electrons in the other orbitals spin in opposite directions and magnetically cancel each other. The unpaired electron, however, creates a magnetic field. Electron spin resonance is a method of detecting changes of spin in unpaired electrons in a powerful magnetic field that are exposed to microwave radio signals, much in the manner of the MRI scanner (the magnetic resonance imaging scanner is the successor to the CT scanner and produced stunning resolution down the the finest detail).

The powerful magnetic field is produced by massive superconducting magnets in the scanner. This causes the atoms to take up an orientation along the lines or force of the field, but facing in one or other direction. Small radio signals of a frequency equal to that of the spin resonance of the atoms are now applied. This causes some of the atoms to flip from facing one way to facing the other way. After the radio signal ceases, they flip back and in so doing emit their own small radio signals. These are detected by the machine. The location of their sources can be computed and a picture built up.

Isn't it possible that free radicals are just a by-product of other much more important disease processes going on in the body?
It's possible. But even the little that is known today about free radicals answers a great many questions that could not be answered before. That knowledge is consistent with a lot of established facts. There is a principle in logic, highly regarded by medical and other scientists, called Occam's razor. This states that a single explanation that accounts for many apparently unrelated facts is more likely to be right than a lot of different explanations. Unifying principles of this kind have been immensely fruitful throughout the history of science. I rather suspect that this is going to be another one.

Antioxidant Vitamins in Food

This appendix is not intended to imply that you can get all the antioxidants you need from your diet. Also, I would like to make the point that vitamins C and E are not, in some mysterious way, 'better' when you get them from natural foods than from a bottle. Ascorbic acid synthesized in a factory and supplied in a pill is *exactly identical* to ascorbic acid from broccoli. Neither offers any advantage over the other. The same goes for tocopherol. In chemistry, a synthetic substance is not a second-grade substitute for the real thing. It *is* the real thing.

These things being said, there is every reason to try to ensure that your diet is as high as it reasonably can be in antioxidant vitamins. These lists will help you to achieve that.

Vitamin C

Comparative amounts in various foods:

Very high C content
Blackcurrants, sweet red and green peppers, broccoli spears, parsley, kale, hot chili peppers.

High C content
Cabbage, Brussels sprouts, cauliflower, chives, collard cabbages, mustard greens.

Intermediate C content
Oranges, limes, lemons, strawberries, ripe tomatoes, cantaloupe, chicory, asparagus, artichokes, fennel, radishes, spinach.

Comparatively low C content
All other fruit. Carrots, celery, corn, cucumber, bamboo shoots, garlic, horse radish, potatoes, onions, rhubarb, parsnips, green tomatoes.

Vitamin E

This vitamin is a fat-soluble substance and is widely distributed in foodstuffs. Whatever your diet, it is very hard to get so little that you suffer deficiency of the vitamin. Only people with an absorption disorder are liable to become deficient in vitamin E.

High E sources
The richest sources are seed germ oils such as sunflower oil, palm oil and walnut oil, wheat germ, lettuce and alfalfa.

Other E sources
The vitamin is present in all vegetable oils, vegetable suet, margarine, nuts, peas, beans and other legumes, leafy green vegetables, cereals generally, milk, butter, animal fats, liver,

meat, fish, poultry and egg yolk.

Margarine has at least 13 times as much vitamin E as butter, and, weight for weight, a salmon steak contains about 10 times as much vitamin E as a beefsteak. The more polyunsaturated fats you eat, the more vitamin E you will get. Polyunsaturated fats stay liquid at room temperature. In general, they are vegetable rather than animal fats.

Glossary

acne a common skin disease of adolescence and early adult life, affecting white people and featuring blackheads, pimples and scarring.

addiction dependence on the repeated use of a drug such as nicotine, alcohol or heroin for comfort of mind or body.

aflatoxin a poison produced by the fungus *Aspergillus flavus* which grows on peanuts and grains stored in damp conditions, and which can cause liver cancer.

AIDS the acquired immune deficiency syndrome, caused by the human immunodeficiency virus (HIV).

aldehyde any organic compound containing the group -CHO (one atom each of carbon, hydrogen and oxygen).

alpha-tocopherol vitamin E.

anaemia a reduction in the amount of the oxygen-carrying substance haemoglobin in the blood.

aneurysm a berry-like or diffuse swelling on an artery, usually at or near a branch, caused by weakness in the artery wall, commonly from atherosclerosis.

angina pectoris the symptom of oppression, pain or tightness in the centre of the chest which occurs when the coronary arteries are unable to provide an adequate blood supply to meet the demands of the heart muscle.

angiography a form of X-ray examination using a fluid opaque to X-rays which renders the blood visible in blood vessels into which it has been injected.

antioxidant a substance capable of preventing the oxidation of organic molecules; a substance, such as vitamin C or vitamin E, capable of 'mopping up' damaging free radicals.

aorta the main artery of the body that arises directly from the heart and supplies branches to all parts.

aromatic hydrocarbon an organic compound containing a ring of six carbon atoms joined by alternating single and double bonds.

artery an elastic, muscular-walled tube carrying blood at high pressure from the heart to any part of the body.

atherosclerosis a degenerative disease of arteries in which fatty plaques develop on the inner lining of arteries so that the normal flow of blood is impeded. It is the major cause of death in the Western world and is responsible for more deaths than any other single condition.

atom the smallest quantity of an element that can take part in a chemical reaction.

balloon angioplasty the use of a balloon catheter to restore more normal width to an artery narrowed by atherosclerosis.

balloon catheter	a fine double tube, with an expandable cylindrical inflatable portion near one end, that can be passed along an artery to an area partially blocked by disease and inflated so as to crush the atherosclerotic plaque into the wall and widen the vessel.
benign	not malignant; mild, not usually tending to cause death.
beta-carotene	the orange pigment in carrots and other vegetables that is converted to vitamin A by the liver. It is a powerful antioxidant.
BHA	see butylated hydroxyanisole
BHT	see butylated hydroxytoluene
bile duct	the tube leading from the liver to the intestine down which bile passes.
bonds	the chemical linkages between atoms joining to form molecules.
brain damage	any permanent loss of full brain function, however caused.
bronchiole	one of the small air tubes of the lungs.
butyl-alpha-phenylnitrone	an antioxidant substance that has been used experimentally to prevent free radical damage.
BPN	see butyl-alpha-phenylnitrone.
butylated hydroxyanisole	an antioxidant widely used as a food preservative.
butylated hydroxytoluene	an antioxidant widely used as a food preservative.
calcification	the laying down of chalky material in living tissues.

115

carbonyl group	a cluster consisting of a linked carbon and oxygen atom.
carcinogen	anything that can cause cancer.
carcinoma	a cancer of surface cells — the commonest class of cancers.
carotenoids	a group of pigments related to vitamin A.
carotid	one of the two main arteries on the side of the neck that carry blood up to the brain.
catalase	an enzyme that breaks down hydrogen peroxide into water and oxygen.
cataract	any opacification of the internal lens of the eye.
cell	the structural and function unit of all living things.
cerebral haemorrhage	bleeding into the brain.
ceruloplasmin	one of the body's natural antioxidants.
chemical reaction	any process in which atoms form linkages or separate.
chemistry	the science of the composition, properties and reactions of substances.
cholesterol	an essential fatty substance found in all body tissues, especially in cell membranes, that is also used by the body to synthesize other steroid substances.
compound	a substance containing atoms of two or more elements held together by chemical bonds.
congenital malformation	any bodily abnormality present at birth.

conjunctiva	the transparent membrane that covers the white of the eye and the inside of the eyelids.
contact inhibition	the restraint on cell reproduction caused by contact with adjacent cells.
cornea	the transparent front lens of the eye.
coronary arteries	the two arteries that arise from the aorta and divide to form branches that spread over the surface of the heart to supply the constantly contracting muscle with blood.
coronary thrombosis	clotting of blood in a coronary artery of the heart, almost always at the site of an atherosclerotic plaque.
crystalline lens	the internal lens of the eye that lies just behind the coloured iris.
cysteine	a sulphur-containing amino acid (protein building-block).
D-penicillamine	one of the body's natural antioxidants.
dementia	progressive loss of mind, commonly the result of atherosclerosis of the arteries supplying the brain.
dermatologist	a skin specialist.
detoxication	a chemical change that renders a poisonous substance safer.
DNA	deoxyribonucleic acid, the double-helix molecule that contains the genetic code blueprint for the structure of all the body proteins.
dopamine	an important chemical found in the brain that can carry information and that is used to form adrenaline.

Dupuytren's contracture	a tightening of the fibrous layer below the skin of the palm of the hand so that the fingers are left permanently bent.
electron	the tiny negatively-charged particle on the outside of atoms that forms the linkages in chemical bonds and whose unbalanced presence forms a free radical.
electron paramagnetic resonance spectroscopy	an advanced technique for detecting the presence of free radicals.
element	one of the 92 naturally occurring substances of which the universe is made. Elements contain only one kind of atom and cannot be broken down further by chemical means.
empirical treatment	treatment without an explanatory basis.
emulsifier	any agent that allows oil and water to mix thoroughly to form a milky liquid.
endonuclease	an enzyme that can cut DNA at any point.
enzyme	a protein capable of greatly accelerating the rate of an organic chemical reaction.
epidermis	the outer layer of the skin.
epithelium	a layer of cells, covering any internal or external surface of the body, that prevents body tissues from healing together.
exonucleases	enzymes that can cut a length of DNA from a free end.
fetus	the human embryo from about the second month of pregnancy to the time of birth.
fibroblasts	cells that form the collagen protein fibrous tissue.

flavonoids	a group of organic compounds that form the colouring matter of plants and flowers.
free radicals	an atom or group of atoms with an unpaired electron, forming a chemically highly active agent avid to latch on to any nearby molecule and to oxidize it. Free radicals are so active that most of them exist only for very short periods before being inactivated on attacking another molecule. In so doing, however, they can convert the second molecule into a free radical and thus start a damaging chain reaction.
French paradox	the surprisingly low incidence of athero-sclerosis in a population with a high dietary intake of saturated fats.
gangrene	death of tissue.
gerontology	the science of ageing.
glucose	a simple sugar, the main fuel of the body.
glucose-6-phosphate dehydrogenase	an enzyme important in carbohydrate usage in the body. Deficiency causes a form of anaemia.
glutathione	one of the body's natural antioxidants.
heart attack	death of a segment of the heart muscle as a result of coronary thrombosis or coronary spasm.
heart failure	the point at which the heart is no longer able to keep the blood circulating adequately, so that stagnation occurs with fluid accumulation in the tissues.
high-density lipoproteins	complexes of fats and proteins, with a preponderance of the latter, that move from the body tissues to the liver.

HIV positive | having antibodies to the human immuno-deficiency virus.

hormones | chemical messengers that help to control and co-ordinate various body and cellular functions.

hydrogen peroxide | a molecule similar to that of water but containing an additional oxygen atom so that it is a strong oxidizing agent.

hydroxyl ion | one of the two parts into which the water molecule naturally splits.

hydroxyl radical | a highly active free radical consisting of a hydrogen atom and an oxygen atom with a single unpaired electron.

hypoxanthine | a substance formed when nucleoproteins (proteins bound to nucleic acid) are broken down, as by free radicals.

inflammation | the body's response to injury. Local blood supply increases and cells of the immune system, such as phagocytes, are brought to the site.

intravenous | within a vein.

ion | an electrically charged atom or group of atoms formed when an electron is gained or lost.

iris | the coloured part of the eye with a central hole, the pupil.

junk DNA | DNA that does not carry genetic information.

LDLS | see low-density lipoproteins.

lentigines | large age-related freckles on the skin. The singular is lentigo.

leukaemia	a kind of cancer of the blood-forming tissues in the bone marrow in which a great excess of abnormal white blood cells is produced so that the blood cannot properly perform its vital functions.
lipids	fats.
liver	the main site of biochemical activity in the body.
low-density lipoproteins	complexes of fats and proteins, with a preponderance of the former, that move from the liver to the body tissues.
malignancy	having a tendency to cause death or serious bodily disorder.
malignant melanoma	a cancer of the skin colouring cells, the melanocytes.
malonaldehyde	a substance released in the course of high levels of tissue oxidation and thus serving as a marker of free radical activity.
metabolic rate	the speed with which the bodily chemical processes occur.
metabolism	the totality of the chemical processes occurring in the body and resulting in growth, tissue breakdown, the production of energy, the disposal of unwanted substances, and so on. Metabolism includes build-up (anabolism) and breakdown (catabolism).
metastasis	remote spread of cancer by seeding out of small groups of cancer cells conveyed by the blood or the lymph.
micrometastases	inapparent transmission of microscopic groups of cancer cells.
micronuclei	fragments of DNA released into the cell

fluids after free radical and other damage.

mitochondria	small spherical or rod-like bodies in cells that contain enzymes responsible for energy production.
molecule	the smallest unit of a chemical compound, consisting of two or more atoms bound together by chemical bonds. Some molecules, such as those of protein, are very large.
mutation	a change in DNA that damages or alters its genetic effect.
naphthols	a group of antioxidant substances.
night blindness	poor vision in dim light, as occurs in vitamin A deficiency.
nitrosamines	a class of oily compounds containing the group $=NNO$. They are able to cause cancer.
oesophagus	the gullet, down which food passes to the stomach.
oncogenes	genes that can activate DNA in such a way as to turn the cell cancerous.
osteomalacia	softening of the bones in adults from calcium deficiency secondary to vitamin D deficiency.
oxidation	the process of undergoing a combination with oxygen or of suffering a loss of electrons. Oxidation is usually damaging, as in rusting or burning, but is an essential part of the process of releasing energy in the body and elsewhere.
oxidative stress	a term widely used to refer to the action of free radicals.
paediatrician	a specialist in child medicine.

peroxidation	a chemical reaction, stimulated in the body by poisons and infections, in which oxygen atoms are freed and then attached to molecules such as that of water to form substances capable of strong oxidation.
phagocytes	scavenging cells of the immune system that engulf and destroy germs and unwanted material by forming free radicals.
phenol	carbolic acid, one of a class of compounds containing a benzene ring and a hydroxyl group.
phenolic	containing, or derived from, phenol.
photo-ageing	the damaging effect on skin of long-term exposure to light.
plaques	the term used for the raised mounds of degenerate muscle cells and cholesterol that from on the inner lining of arteries in the disease of atherosclerosis.
polyunsaturated fats	fats containing fatty acids in which many of the carbon linkages have double bonds and are thus more easily broken than the more stable single bonds. Unsaturated fats are usually liquid at room temperature.
progeria	a rare disease in which the ageing of a lifetime occurs in the first ten years or so of life.
prospective studies	trials, as of the value of antioxidant supplements, in which the conditions are set before the trials begin and the results are assessed in the future.
protein	the main constructional and functional material of the body, formed by the linkage of various combinations of 20 amino acids into large molecules. Proteins may be soluble, as in the case of the blood proteins,

antibodies and enzymes, or insoluble, as in the case of the collagen of bones and connective tissue and the keratin of the hair and nails.

radical

a chemical group or associated cluster of atoms usually forming a part of a molecule that often retains its identity in the course of chemical reactions.

reperfusion

the renewed flow of blood into an area of the body after it has been cut off. This results from the opening up of nearby closed blood vessels and is commonly associated with intense free radicals action.

replication

the process of exact copying, as occurs in DNA before cell reproduction.

retinol

vitamin A.

retrolental fibroplasia

a serious and often blinding eye disorder occurring in premature babies given too much oxygen.

rickets

bone softening and distortion occurring in infants deficient in vitamin D.

saturated fat

fat containing fatty acids whose carbon atom linkages are all by single, and thus stable, bonds. Most saturated fats are solid at room temperature.

scurvy

the bleeding disorder from defective synthesis of collagen caused by a deficiency of vitamin C.

seminal fluid

the sticky fluid containing millions of sperms that is emitted during sexual ejaculation.

solar radiation

radiation from the sun, of which the most biologically damaging wavelengths are in the ultraviolet part of the spectrum.

stroke	a serious disorder resulting from brain damage caused by deprivation of blood or bleeding into or around the brain.
substantia nigra	a darkly-pigmented part of the brain that produces the substance dopamine.
superoxide	a metal oxide containing an oxygen ion. One of the most important free radicals formed in the body, one that can attack fats, proteins and carbohydrates.
superoxide dismutase	one of the body's natural antioxidants, capable of inactivating the superoxide free radical.
telangiectasis	'broken veins'.
telomeres	the end segments of the DNA of chromosomes.
thrombosis	clotting of blood within an artery or a vein.
TIA	see transient ischaemic attack.
tissue	any collection of joined cells.
tissue culture	the artificial growth of sheets of body cells, such as fibroblasts, in glass dishes in the laboratory.
tocopherol	vitamin E.
tocopherols	a group of compounds related to or constituting vitamin E.
transferrin	one of the body's natural antioxidants.
transient ischaemic attack	a mini-stroke lasting for less than 24 hours. TIAs are serious warnings that a full stroke, with permanent damage, may occur at any time.

tretinoin	the active form of vitamin A in all body tissues except the retina of the eye.
ulceration	a breakdown of any body surface to form a crater and expose the underlying tissue.
ultraviolet light	the part of the electromagnetic spectrum that lies between visible light and X-rays. Most of the sun's UVL is filtered out by the atmosphere, but it is still capable of provoking much free radical formation in the skin.
ultraviolet radiation	see ultraviolet light.
unstable angina	angina pectoris that shows a tendency to worsen.
xanthine	a substance involved in the production of free radicals, that can act as a marker of free radical activity.

Index

THE ANTIOXIDANT RECIPE BOOK

Concentrating on practical, everyday meals which
are rich in vitamins C, E and betacarotene,
The Antioxicant Recipe Book is the first cookery book
of its kind.

Alongside a simple account of how a high antioxidant
diet can counter the damaging effects of free radicals,
Amanda Ursell, nutritional consultant and presenter of
the Channel 4 series "Eat Up", transforms theory
into practice with a guide to the Top 20 Antioxidant
Superfoods and over 100 tempting recipe
suggestions for:

- breakfasts
- light and main meals
- packed lunches
- drinks